# Lecture Notes of the Institute for Computer Sciences, Social Informatics and Telecommunications Engineering   207

More information about this series at http://www.springer.com/series/8197

Nuria Oliver · Silvia Serino
Aleksandar Matic · Pietro Cipresso
Nenad Filipovic · Liljana Gavrilovska (Eds.)

# Pervasive Computing Paradigms for Mental Health

Selected Papers from MindCare 2016
Fabulous 2016, and IIoT 2015

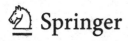 Springer

*Editors*
Nuria Oliver
Vodafone Research
Barcelona
Spain

Silvia Serino
Catholic University of Milan
Milan
Italy

Aleksandar Matic
Telefónica
Barcelona
Spain

Pietro Cipresso
3 Piano-Endocrinologia
Istituto Auxologico Italiano
Milan
Italy

Nenad Filipovic
University of Kragujevac
Kragujevac
Serbia

Liljana Gavrilovska
Ss. Cyril and Methodius University
    in Skopje
Skopje
Macedonia

ISSN 1867-8211          ISSN 1867-822X   (electronic)
Lecture Notes of the Institute for Computer Sciences, Social Informatics
and Telecommunications Engineering
ISBN 978-3-319-74934-1          ISBN 978-3-319-74935-8   (eBook)
https://doi.org/10.1007/978-3-319-74935-8

Library of Congress Control Number: 2018934325

Printed on acid-free paper

This Springer imprint is published by the registered company Springer International
Publishing AG part of Springer Nature
The registered company address is: Gewerbestrasse 11, 6330 Cham, Switzerland

# Preface

The 2016 International Symposium on Pervasive Computing Paradigms for Mental Health – MindCare was held in Barcelona, Spain, during November 28–29, 2016.

The symposium discussed the use of innovative technologies in favor of maintaining and improving psychological well-being and it brought together the community of researchers and practitioners from different domains, including technology, psychiatry, and psychology.

MindCare in its six editions has gathered scientists from more than 30 countries allowing for the creation of a truly multidisciplinary community that shares a common interest and passion for advancing the state of the art by building new paradigms in mental health care.

MindCare 2016 in Barcelona covered a diverse set of topics and featured several cutting-edge technologies, from video and audio technologies to VR and wearable computing.

The two keynote speakers, Prof. Jakob Bardram and Dr. Aureli Soria-Frisch, shared the learnings from practical implementation of their latest research studies, in using mobile technologies for monitoring bipolar disorder and in using VR for treating various mental health problems, respectively.

In addition, the proceedings include the papers from the FABULOUS 2016 Workshop, which took place in Belgrade, Serbia, during October 24–26, 2016.

Nuria Oliver
Silvia Serino
Aleksandar Matic
Pietro Cipresso
Nenad Filipovic
Liljana Gavrilovska

# Organization

## Steering Committee

### Steering Committee Chair

Imrich Chlamtac            Create-Net, Italy

### Technological Perspectives Chair

Anind K. Dey            Carnegie Mellon University, USA

### Psychological Perspectives Chair

Giuseppe Riva            Istituto Auxologico Italiano, Italy

## Organizing Committee

### General Chairs

Nuria Oliver            Telefonica I+D, Spain
Silvia Serino            Catholic University of Milan, Italy
Aleksandar Matic            Telefonica I+D, Spain
Pietro Cipresso            Istituto Auxologico Italiano, Italy

### Program Chairs

Nervo Verdezoto            University of Leicester, UK
David Coyle            University College Dublin, Ireland

### Publication Chair

Ana Tajadura-Jimenez            University College London, UK

### Poster Chairs

Elisa Pedroli            Istituto Auxologico Italiano, Italy
Mirjana Prpa            School of Interactive Arts + Technology (SIAT), Canada

### Publicity Chairs

Ivan Alsina Jurnet            Universitat de Vic - Universitat Central de Catalunya, Spain
Diego Hidalgo Mazzei            Hospital Clinic, Barcelona, Spain

## Technical Program Committee

| | |
|---|---|
| Afsaneh Doryab | Carnegie Mellon University, USA |
| Anja Thieme | Microsoft Research Cambridge, UK |
| Anouk Keizer | Utrecht University, The Netherlands |
| Conor Linehan | University of Cork, Ireland |
| Erik Grönvall | IT University of Copenhagen, Denmark |
| Francesca Morganti | University of Bergamo, Italy |
| Francisco Nunes | Universidade Nova de Lisboa, Portugal |
| Javier Hernandez | MIT Media Lab, USA |
| Jean Marcel Dos Reis Costa | Cornell University, USA |
| José Gutiérrez-Maldonado | Universidad de Barcelona, Spain |
| Julian Childs | Anna Freud Centre, UK |
| Katarzyna Wac | University of Copenhagen, Denmark |
| Mads Frost | IT University of Copenhagen, Denmark |
| Maria Angela Ferrario | Lancaster University, UK |
| Maria Wolters | University of Edinburgh, UK |
| Mariano Alcaniz | Laboratorio de Neurotecnologías Inmersivas |
| Mark Matthews | University of Cornell, USA |
| Pedro Gamito | Universidade Lusófona, Portugal |
| Rosa Banos | Universitat de València, Spain |
| Stefano Triberti | Università Cattolica di Milano, Italy |
| Willem-Paul Brinkman | Delft University of Technology, The Netherlands |

# Workshop: FABULOUS 2016 Conference Organization

## Steering Committee

| | |
|---|---|
| Imrich Chlamtac | Create-Net and University of Trento, Italy |
| Liljana Gavrilovska | Ss. Cyril and Methodius University in Skopje, Macedonia |
| Alberto Leon-Garcia | University of Toronto, Canada |

## Organizing Committee

### General Chair

Nenad Filipovic — University of Kragujevac, Serbia

### General Co-chairs

| | |
|---|---|
| Liljana Gavrilovska | Ss. Cyril and Methodius University in Skopje, Macedonia |
| Veljko Milutinovic | University of Belgrade, Serbia |

### Technical Program Committee Chair

Dalibor Nikolic — University of Kragujevac, Serbia

### Web Chair

Djordje Dimitrijevic — University of Kragujevac, Serbia

### Publications Chair

Velibor Isailovic — University of Kragujevac, Serbia

### Publicity and Social Media Chair

Milena Djordjevic — University of Kragujevac, Serbia

### Workshops Chair

Aleksandar Peulic — University of Kragujevac, Serbia

### Sponsorship and Exhibits Chair

Neda Vidanovic — University of Kragujevac, Serbia

### Local Chair

Milica Kaplarevic — University of Kragujevac, Serbia

**Conference Manager**

Anna Horvathova            EAI - European Alliance for Innovation

## Technical Program Committee

| | |
|---|---|
| Ian Akyildiz | Georgia Institute of Technology, Atlanta, GA, USA |
| Bojana Andjelkovic Cirkovic | University of Kragujevac, Serbia |
| Vladimir Atanasovski | Ss. Cyril and Methodius University in Skopje, Macedonia |
| Zoran Babovic | University of Belgrade, Serbia |
| Nikolaos Bourbakis | Wright State University, OH, USA |
| Hakan Delic | Bogaziçi University, Turkey |
| Luca De Nardis | Sapienza University of Rome, Italy |
| Daniel Denkovski | Ss. Cyril and Methodius University in Skopje, Macedonia |
| Themis Exarchos | FORTH |
| Nenad Filipovic | University of Kragujevac, Serbia |
| Dimitris Fotiadis | University of Ioannina, Greece |
| Octavian Fratu | University POLITEHNICA of Bucharest, Romania |
| Ada Gavrilovska | Georgia Tech, GA, USA |
| Liljana Gavrilovska | Ss. Cyril and Methodius University in Skopje, Macedonia |
| Mohamed Ghalwash | SERC |
| Andrea Giorgetti | University of Bologna, Italy |
| Velibor Isailovic | University of Kragujevac, Serbia |
| Milos Ivanovic | University of Kragujevac, Serbia |
| Vladisav Jelisavcic | Mathematical Institute SANU, Serbia |
| Emil Jovanov | The University of Alabama in Huntsville, AL, USA |
| Anton Kos | Ljubljana University, Slovenia |
| Sofoklis Kyriazakos | Aalborg University, Denmark |
| Miodrag Manic | University of Nis, Serbia |
| Miodrag Mihaljevic | Mathematical Institute SANU, Serbia |
| Zarko Milosevic | University of Kragujevac, Serbia |
| Miljan Milosevic | University of Kragujevac, Serbia |
| Veljko Milutinovic | University of Belgrade, Serbia |
| Onur Mutlu | Carnegie Mellon University, PA, USA |
| Dalibor Nikolic | University of Kragujevac, Serbia |
| Zoran Obradovic | Temple University |
| Aleksandar Peulic | University of Kragujevac, Serbia |
| Petar Popovski | Aalborg University, Denmark |
| Vladimir Poulkov | Technical University in Sofia, Bulgaria |
| Milos Radovic | University of Kragujevac, Serbia |

| | |
|---|---|
| Valentin Rakovic | Ss. Cyril and Methodius University in Skopje, Macedonia |
| Vesna Rankovic | University of Kragujevac, Serbia |
| Igor Saveljic | University of Kragujevac, Serbia |
| Hans-Peter Schwefel | FTW |
| Huseyin Seker | Northumbria University, UK |
| Boban Stojanovic | University of Kragujevac, Serbia |
| Dimitar Trajanov | Ss. Cyril and Methodius University in Skopje, Macedonia |
| Miroslav Trajanovic | University of Nis, Serbia |
| Jaap van de Beek | Luleå University of Technology, Sweden |
| Arso Vukicevic | University of Kragujevac, Serbia |
| Arda Yurdakul | Boğaziçi University, Turkey |
| Vladimir Zlokolica | University of Novi Sad, Serbia |

# Contents

## FABULOUS 2016

## IIoT 2015

## Short Papers

MindCare 2016

# Computer-Based Programs as Suitable Intervention Tools for Older People with Mental Disorders

Blanka Klimova[(✉)]

Faculty of Informatics and Management, University of Hradec Kralove,
Rokitanskeho 62, 500 03 Hradec Kralove, Czech Republic
blanka.klimova@uhk.cz

**Abstract.** Currently, there is no reliable cure for mental disorder such as depression. However, there are a few strategies which can help in the treatment of their symptoms. These comprise both pharmacological and non-pharmacological approaches. The purpose of this article is to discuss the role of the Internet and computer-based programs as an appropriate intervention tool for older adults with depression. This is done by conducting a literature search in the databases Web of Science, Scopus, MEDLINE and Springer, and consequently by evaluating the findings of the relevant studies. Based on the findings, computer-based programs targeted at older people with depression may be beneficial in several ways: they are non-invasive treatments, they can be tailored-made to older people's needs, they are cost-effective and can be made widely available, and they appear to be an effective intervention tool, especially as far as the short-term effects are concerned. Nevertheless, it is important to pay close attention to the methodological standards in future clinical studies, as well as to the efficacy of these computer-based programs aimed at older individuals with depression.

**Keywords:** Depression · Computer-based programs · The internet
Older people · Intervention · Review

## 1 Introduction

Current trends indicate that there is an increasing number of older population groups. In fact, in the year of 2000, older people aged 65+ represented 12.4% of the entire population. In 2030 this number is expected to rise to 19% and by the year of 2050 it should reach 22% [1]. Over 20% of adults aged 60+ suffer from a mental or neurological disorder (excluding headache disorders) [2]. One of the most common neuropsychiatric disorders among older people is depression.

Depression is usually defined as a mood disorder that causes a constant feeling of sadness and loss of interest and pleasure. Other main symptoms comprise feelings of guilt or low self-esteem, disturbed sleep or appetite, feelings of tiredness and poor concentration. Depression can affect patient´s life persistently or just in waves. In severe cases, it can result in suicide [3]. In case of older people, these symptoms are often overlooked and untreated because they coincide with other problems older people

N. Oliver et al. (Eds.): MindCare 2016/Fabulous 2016/IIoT 2015, LNICST 207, pp. 3–9, 2018.
https://doi.org/10.1007/978-3-319-74935-8_1

may have. Moreover, this mental disorder is quite serious since it can lead to great suffering and impaired functioning in daily life, especially cognitive functioning.

At present, however, there is no reliable cure for this disorder, but there are a few strategies which can help in the treatment of its symptoms. These comprise both pharmacological and non-pharmacological approaches [4]. Most recently, with the emergence of information and communication technologies (ICT), especially the Internet and computer-based programs started to be used as suitable intervention tools among older people with depression. This is also caused by the fact that older people have relatively easy access to computers [5]. In addition, the generation of the so-called baby boomers approaching retirement is fairly comfortable using ICT [6] although research shows that these older adults are higher-income and more educated seniors [7]. Recent research studies also reveal that there is a significant increase in the use of ICT, especially the Internet and computer-based programs, for health purposes [8–11].

The aim of this article is to discuss the role of the Internet and computer-based programs as an appropriate intervention tool for older adults with depression.

## 2 Methods

The methodology of this review article follows Moher et al. [12] and Kurz and Baelen [13]. The The main method was a systematic review whose aim was to find the research studies on the basis of the key words in four databases: Web of Science, Springer, Scopus, and MEDLINE. This review was conducted in the period from 2010 to 2015 for the following key words: *computer* AND *mental disorder* AND *aging*; and *computer* AND *depression* AND *aging*. Altogether 423 studies were found via the database search and 22 studies via other sources, which included conference proceedings and books outside the scope of the databases described above. After a thorough review of the titles, duplication and abstracts of the selected studies, only 23 studies remained for the full-text analysis. After that, only five clinical studies were detected. The study was included if it matched the corresponding period, i.e., from 2010 up to 2015. The selection period starts with the year of 2010 since this is the year when the clinical trials conducted among older adults started to appear due to the fact that older individuals began to be more digitally literate and able to use the Internet on a daily basis [14]. Thus, the study was included if it matched the corresponding period, i.e., from 2010 up to 2015; if it involved older people with depression (mild to moderate depression), and focused on the use of the Internet, and/or computer-based programs. The remaining selected theoretical articles, review articles and book chapters were used in the part on discussion and in the introduction for the exploration of the research topic and comparison of findings.

## 3 Findings

Altogether five clinical studies are described in the following Table 1. Out of these five clinical studies, three are randomized controlled trials, one is a clinical trial and one is a pilot study. All of them deal with older people who suffer from mild to moderate depression. Therefore the research studies which were not exclusively focused on the research topic, were reviews, or concentrated on healthy older individuals, e.g., [15, 16] were excluded. All five clinical studies are summarized in alphabetical order of their first author in Table 1 below.

**Table 1.** Overview of the clinical studies on the use of computer-based programs for older people with depression.

| Study | Type of intervention | No. of subjects | Intervention period | Findings | Limitations |
|---|---|---|---|---|---|
| Dear et al. [17] CT | iCBT | 20 subjects (elevated symptoms of depression) | 5 educational lessons and homework summaries within 8 weeks and 3 weeks of follow-up | Participants improved significantly on the PHQ-9 and Geriatric Depression Scale (GDS), with large within-group effect sizes (Cohen's d) at follow-up of 1.41 and 2.04, respectively | Small sample size; short period; no control group |
| Khatri et al. [18] PS | Online CBT | 18 subjects with diagnostic mental disorders | 13 weeks | The findings show that the online CBT could be delivered in a technology-supported environment (on-line video conferencing) and can meet the same professional practice standards and outcomes as face-to-face delivery | Small sample size; short period |
| Lagana, Garcia [19] RCT | One-to-one computer and Internet training | 60 older people with depression | 6 weeks | There were significant improvements in favor of the experimental group in computer self-efficacy; there was a decreased percentage of significantly depressed experimental subjects from 36.7% at baseline to 16.7% at the end of intervention | Short period; a lack of sample representation |

*(continued)*

**Table 1.** (*continued*)

| Study | Type of intervention | No. of subjects | Intervention period | Findings | Limitations |
|---|---|---|---|---|---|
| Preschl et al. [20] RCT | Life-review therapy with computer supplements | 36 older people with elevated depressive symptoms | 6 weeks | The results indicate that depressive symptoms decreased significantly over time until the three-month follow-up in the intervention group compared to the control group (pre to post: d = 1.13; pre to follow-up: d = 1.27; and group $\times$ time effect pre to post: d = 0.72) | Small sample size; short period |
| Titov et al. [21] RCT | iCBT | 27 subjects in the intervention group and 25 subjects in the control group, all older than 60 years | 8 weeks | The findings show considerably lower scores on the PHQ-9 (Cohen's $d$ = 2.08; 95% CI: 1.38 – 2.72) and on a measure of anxiety (Generalized Anxiety Disorder-7 Item) (Cohen's $d$ = 1.22; 95% CI: 0.61–1.79) in the intervention group compared to the control group at posttreatment | Small sample size; short period |

Source: author's own processing

Explanation: CBT - Cognitive Behavior Therapy; CS – cohort study; CT – clinical trial; iCBT - Internet-delivered Cognitive Behavior Therapy; PS – pilot study; RCT – randomized controlled trial

## 4  Discussion

The results of the clinical studies described above indicate that computer-based programs appear to be good intervention tools for older people with depression. Generally, the Internet or web-based interventions have been shown to deliver efficacious psychological intervention programs for depression on a large scale [22]. Especially the online cognitive behavior therapist programs, which are evidence-based, time-limited collaborative forms of psychotherapy, seem to be effective [17, 18, 21] and they seem to meet at least the same professional practice standards and outcomes as face-to-face delivery [18]. In addition, these therapist programs are cost-effective and particularly suitable for those having difficulties accessing such services in person [18]. Further-more, Cotton et al. [23] argue that the Internet use may not only contribute to the reduction of symptoms of depression, but also to the decrease of social isolation and loneliness of older people. The decreased loneliness is also supported by the meta-analytic study [24] whose authors examined the effectiveness of computer and Internet training interventions intended to reduce loneliness and depression in older adults. The effect size for loneliness from their five analyzed studies was statistically significant ($Z = 2.085$, $p = 0.037$).

Nevertheless, the last described study [24] and other research studies [25] indicate that there is no efficacy of computer-based programs on depressive symptomatology among older individuals. This is connected with the fact that there are important differences in methodologies used in the clinical trials. Methodological issues such as the use of passive control groups or the failure to consider baseline differences between the groups may lead to overestimation of the training effects, seriously threatening the validity of the findings [26–28].

## 5  Conclusion

Based on the findings of this review article, computer-based programs targeted at older people with depression may be beneficial in several ways: they are non-invasive treatments, they can be tailored-made to older people's needs, they are cost-effective and can be made widely available, and they appear to be an effective intervention tool, especially as far as the short-term effects are concerned. Nevertheless, it is important to pay close attention to the methodological standards in future clinical studies, as well as the efficacy of these computer-based programs aimed at older individuals with depression.

**Acknowledgments.** The paper is supported by the project Excellence (2016/17) at the Faculty of Informatics and Management of the University of Hradec Kralove, Czech Republic.

## References

1. Transgenerational Design Matters. The Demographics of Aging. http://transgenerational.org/aging/demographics.htm
2. WHO: http://www.who.int/mediacentre/factsheets/fs381/en/
3. WHO: Depression: Definition. http://www.euro.who.int/en/health-topics/noncommunicable-diseases/pages/news/news/2012/10/depression-in-europe/depression-definition
4. Klimova, B., Maresova, P., Kuca, K.: Non-pharmacological approaches to the prevention and treatment of alzheimer's disease with respect to the rising treatment costs. Curr. Alzheimer Res. **13**(11), 1249–1258 (2016)
5. Heart, T., Kalderon, E.: Older adults: are they ready to adopt health-related ICT? Int. J. Med. Informatics **82**, e209–e231 (2013)
6. Virginia Assistive Technology System: Assistive Technology and Aging. A Handbook for Virginians Who Are Aging and Their Caregivers. http://www.vda.virginia.gov/pdfdocs/Assistive%20Technology%20&%20Aging%20-%20All.pdf

7. Smith, A.: Older Adults and Technology Use. http://www.pewinternet.org/2014/04/03/older-adults-and-technology-use/

8. Bujnowska-Fedak, M.M.: Trends in the use of the internet for health purposes in Poland. BMC **15**, 194 (2015)

9. Wangberg, S., Andreassen, H., Kummervold, P., Wynn, R., Sørensen, T.: Use of the internet for health purposes: trends in Norway 2000–2010. Scand. J. Caring. Sci. Dic. **23**(4), 691–696 (2009)

10. Siliquini, R., Ceruti, M., Lovato, E., Bert, F., Bruno, S., De Vito, E., et al.: Surfing the internet for health information: An Italian survey use and population choices. BMC Med. Inform. Decis. **11**, 21 (2011)

11. Rockmann, R., Gewald, H.: Elderly people in eHealth: who are they? Procedia Comput. Sci. **63**, 505–510 (2015)

12. Moher, D., Liberati, A., Tetzlaff, J., Altman, D.G.: The PRISMA Group. Preferred reporting items for systematic review and meta-analysis: The PRISMA statement. PLoS Med. **6**(6), e1000097 (2009)

13. Kurz, A., van Baelen, B.: Ginkgo biloba compared with cholinesterase inhibitors in the treatment of dementia: a review based on meta-analyses by the cochrane collaboration. Dement. Geriatr. Cogn. Disord. **18**, 217–226 (2004)

14. Klimova, B., Simonova, I., Poulova, P., Truhlarova, Z., Kuca, K.: Older people and their attitude to the use of information and communication technologies – a review study with special focus on the Czech Republic (older people and their attitude to ICT). Educ. Gerontol. **42**(5), 361–369 (2016)

15. Brunoni, A.R., Boggio, P.S., De Raedt, R., Benseñor, I.M., Lotufo, P.A., Namur, V., et al.: Cognitive control therapy and transcranial direct current stimulation for depression: a randomized, double-blinded controlled trial. J. Affect. Disord. **162**, 43–49 (2014)

16. Morimoto, S.S., Wexler, B.E., Liu, J., Hu, W., Seirup, J., Alexopoulos, G.S.: Neuroplasticity-based computerized cognitive remediation for treatment-resistant geriatric depression. Nature Commun. **5**, 4579 (2014)

17. Dear, B.F., Zou, J., Titov, N., Lorian, C., Johnston, L., Spence, J., et al.: Internet-delivered cognitive behavioural therapy for depression: a feasibility open trial for older adults. Aust. N. Z. J. Psychiatry **47**(2), 169–176 (2013)

18. Khatri, N., Maryiali, E., Tchernikov, I., Shepherd, N.: Comparing telehealth-based and clinic-based group cognitive behavioral therapy for adults with depression and anxiety: a pilot study. Clin. Interv. Aging **9**, 765–770 (2014)

19. Lagana, L., Garcia, J.J.: The mental health impact of computer and internet training on a multi-ethnic sample of community-dwelling older adults: results of a pilot randomized controlled trial. Int. J. Biomed. Sci. **9**(3), 135–147 (2013)

20. Preschl, B., Maercker, A., Wagner, B., Forstmeier, S., Baños, R.M., Alcañiz, M., et al.: Life-review therapy with computer supplements for depression in the elderly: a randomized controlled trial. Aging Ment. Health. **16**(8), 964–974 (2012)

21. Titov, N., Dear, B.F., Ali, S., Zou, J.B., Lorian, C.N., Johnston, L., et al.: Clinical and cost-effectiveness of therapist-guided internet-delivered cognitive behavior therapy for older adults with symptoms of depression: a randomized controlled trial. Behav. Ther. **46**(2), 193–205 (2015)

22. Cockayne, N.L., Glozier, N., Naismith, S.L., Christensen, H., Neal, B., Hickie, I.B.: Internet-based treatment for older adults with depression and co-morbid cardiovascular disease: protocol for a randomised, double-blind, placebo controlled trial. BMC Psychiatry **11**, 10 (2011)

23. Cotten, S.R., Ford, G., Ford, S., Hale, T.M.: Internet use and depression among retired older adults in the United States: a longitudinal analysis. J. Gerontol. B Psychol. Sci. Soc. Sci. **69** (5), 763–771 (2014)
24. Choi, M., Kong, S., Jung, D.: Computer and internet interventions for loneliness and depression in older adults: a meta-analysis. HIR **18**(3), 191–198 (2012)
25. Millán-Calenti, J.C., Lorenzo, T., Núñez-Naveira, L., Buján, A., Rodríguez-Villamil, J.L., Maseda, A.: Efficacy of a computerized cognitive training application on cognition and depressive symptomatology in a group of healthy older adults: a randomized controlled trial. Arch. Gerontol. Geriatr. **61**(3), 337–343 (2015)
26. Melby-Lervåg, M., Hulme, C.: There is no convincing evidence that working memory training is effective: a reply to Au et al. (2014) and Karbach and Verhaeghen (2014). Psychon Bull. Rev. **23**(1), 324–330 (2016)
27. Melby-Lervåg, M., Hulme, C.: Is working memory training effective? a meta-analytic review. Dev. Psychol. **49**(2), 270–291 (2013)
28. Melby-Lervåg, M., Redick, T., Hulme, C.: Working memory training does not improve performance on measures of intelligence or other measures of "far transfer": evidence from a meta-analytic review. Perspect. Psychol. Sci. **11**(4), 512–534 (2016)

# ONParkinson – Innovative mHealth to Support the Triad: Patient, Carer and Health Professional

Rui Neves Madeira[1(✉)] 🆔, Carla Mendes Pereira[2], Sergiu Clipei[2], and Patrícia Macedo[1]

[1] Escola Superior de Tecnologia de Setúbal, IPS, Setúbal, Portugal
{rui.madeira,patricia.macedo}@estsetubal.ips.pt
[2] Escola Superior de Saúde, IPS, Setúbal, Portugal
carla.pereira@ess.ips.pt, sergiu.c3@gmail.com

**Abstract.** The ONParkinson mHealth platform aims to empower an integrated assistance to support end-users of the triad "people with Parkinson's Disease, their carers and health professionals", promoting the self-management in Parkinson's disease. Therefore, ONParkinson is expected to optimize the communication between the triad users, helping them find relevant knowledge to support their clinical issues, as well as allowing the monitoring of patients' daily routine and the recommendation for daily exercises. This mHealth solution was created and materialized after an initial study of the end-users' needs. This paper presents the usability study of the first version of the ONParkinson prototype. According to the usability tests' findings, ONParkinson was perceived by the triad users as easy to use, with functionalities well integrated, useful and attractive. Some recommendations were suggested to enhance its usability, users' satisfaction and continuance intentions.

**Keywords:** Parkinson's disease · mHealth · Mobile computing
Usability · Self-management

## 1 Introduction

Mobile devices can be found everywhere around people, which makes them be seen as a ubiquitous entity, being almost universally connectable and appearing in almost everywhere. Accordingly, there is an emerging consumer-driven demand for a more personalised health system, and there is no question that the rapid evolution of the mobile application market became an important driver for personalisation in the health field. The concept of mHealth is changing how healthcare is delivered [1], with an increased support to the management of chronic diseases [2], such as Parkinson's disease (PD), which is recognised as the most common neurodegenerative disorder after Alzheimer's disease [3, 4], with a higher prevalence in Europe and Portugal [5]. Mobile phones and other networked devices offer a unique opportunity to engage remotely the people involved in managing PD, including both people with PD and health professionals, as well as carers/family.

© ICST Institute for Computer Sciences, Social Informatics and Telecommunications Engineering 2018
N. Oliver et al. (Eds.): MindCare 2016/Fabulous 2016/IIoT 2015, LNICST 207, pp. 10–18, 2018.
https://doi.org/10.1007/978-3-319-74935-8_2

Starting from a study of the needs of the triad "people with PD, their carers and health professionals", our multidisciplinary team proposed the development of an mHealth platform – ONParkinson – based on the empowerment of this triad to help both patients and carers to manage PD better [6]. In this paper, the usability study of the first version of the mHealth prototype is presented.

## 2 Background

Mobile applications (apps) have been designed to support people with PD by providing, for instance, recommendations and instructions about home exercises. However, research findings of its effectiveness are limited. Most studies in this field applied to PD have investigated the use of apps for home-based monitoring and assessment of motor complications with data being used mainly by health professionals for clinical decision [7, 8]. Moreover, more recent studies focused on a user-centred process for the design of apps present positive results. Indeed, findings indicated that people with PD were able to achieve high task completion rates on usability tests, showing that user-centred approaches can be efficient [9].

Furthermore, most of the health services and self-management tools provided have been centred on the person with PD and in supporting clinical decisions. Thus, apps have been developed in order to improve the patients' capabilities of self-management of the PD (e.g., the REMPARK system [9] and the mPower app [10]). However, the involvement of both people with PD and their carers has been highlighted as providing benefits to them [11]. The majority of people with PD live in the community and are cared for by family members, who are often referred to as 'informal' carers that play a vital role, providing social, physical and psychological support over an extended period. The impact of the disease on the lives of people with PD and their carers is wide-ranging, affecting daily living and altering roles. PD is a condition that becomes less predictable over time, with symptoms fluctuating rapidly within the day or week-by-week. The slowness of movement, rigidity, and tremor are often present and will impact on the person's ability to be active. Moreover, there are numerous 'non-motor' symptoms associated with PD, including anxiety, depression, fatigue, pain and sleep disturbance, which are associated with reduced health-related quality of life [3].

Thus, for both the patient and the carer, it is important to understand the disease and its progression in order to manage symptoms and find solutions for their daily challenges, as well as to maintain the communication with health professionals for an effective shared decision-making within the triad. This understanding and symptoms monitoring are expected to increase their ability for self-manage the disease over time, improve their quality of life, reduce carers strain and reduce hospitalization/visits. However, to the best of our knowledge, there are no solutions based on mobile apps in this field aiming to combine both patient and carer's support for a broader management approach of PD.

## 3    ONParkinson

The ONParkinson mHealth solution is a platform formerly known as Smoveen, in which a mobile app is the main interface to provide patients and carers with self-management capabilities to help them feel empowered in their ability to find strategies in a more informed and collaborative way. The mobile device acts as the communication channel between the user and the system. It should remain with the user and it is essential that the user may be able to interact with it as many times as possible. The platform also intends to optimize therapy outside the clinical context with remote support from the health professionals, providing them with an exclusive Web interface.

### 3.1    The Mobile App

The first prototype of this mHealth app was implemented in Java for the Android platform, taking into account that Android apps have the longest reach in the mass market, which give us the intended space to work closely with the ONParkinson's target audience. Although being created to support patients and carers with self-management capabilities within the triad, the "common user" type (user with no account) was considered in the app design. This type of user can install the app and use the open features to consult essential information about PD and ask open questions related to the pathology, without the need of being under the supervision of a health professional registered on the platform.

Considering that the goal of self-management technologies has been to quantify, track, and keep the condition under control [12], this app was designed to provide integrated ways to control the evolution of the disease. It allows the establishment of communication among the triad users, the management of daily tasks (medication and exercises program) and the privileged access to specific information about PD in a simple and natural manner [6]. The concept of ONParkinson has been tested in a first prototype that presents functionalities based on three main dimensions of intervention towards both the patient and the carer (Fig. 1): Information, Calendar and Exercises.

The Information module includes six essential categories from which are commonly asked questions related to PD, namely: "What is Parkinson's Disease?"; "Symptoms"; "Recommendations"; "Caring role"; "Treatments"; and "National legislation".

The Calendar interface presents events regarding medication prescript and exercises program. Usually, these events are inserted in the patient's calendar by the health professional, who use the Web interface to supervise patients' actions. These events cannot be altered either by the patient nor her/his carer(s). Nonetheless, as long as patients have autonomy, they can add events (e.g. medical appointments, treatment sessions, leisure activities or others) to the calendar, as well as can her/his carers, who can also supervise the patients' actions. This approach intends to make the ONParkinson mobile app more comprehensive and useful to the users. The app sends notifications to both the users, patient and carer, as reminders to take the medication or execute the scheduled exercises. This functionality intends to place both the patient and the carer at the centre of the decision, empowering them to manage PD in a more integrated way.

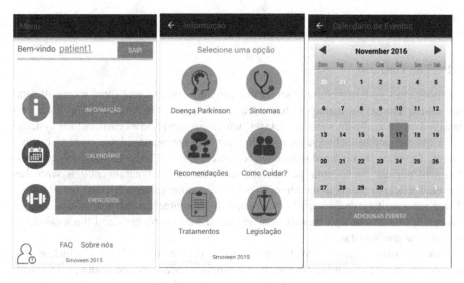

**Fig. 1.** ONParkinson screens: (left) home menu; (middle) information menu; (right) calendar.

The Exercises program interface allows the patient, or the carer, to select generic exercises to follow and learn how to practice them (Fig. 2, left image). Additionally, the user may have a program prescribed by the health professional, which will appear as an event in the calendar. When opening the program, the patient (or the carer in her/his behalf) starts by rating her/his perceived exertion (Borg Scale) (Fig. 2, middle image) and recording the cardiac rate and blood pressure (optional step). Then, the exercises program will initiate, having three distinct phases: warm-up, training and cool

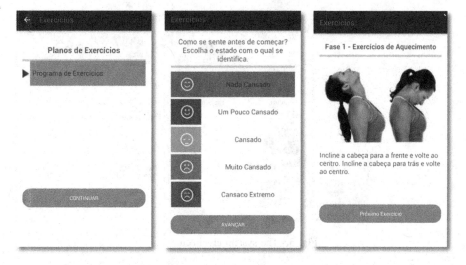

**Fig. 2.** ONParkinson screens: (left) exercises programs; (middle) mood selection; (right) exercise.

down. The right image of Fig. 2 illustrates a warm-up exercise. The session will end up with an evaluation of the perceived exertion, cardiac rate and blood pressure.

## 3.2   The Platform

The platform's system includes a server that contains a central repository where all data are stored. The server manages all the requests from the ONParkinson app instances installed on the end-user's mobile devices, which are identified as clients of the system. All communications between users within the app are managed and synced by the server. The users do not need to be always connected to the Internet to use the app, but this will request connections periodically in order to do synchronizations with the server. The app connects to the server to obtain and store the required data for all users. There are specific synchronization moments to guarantee that all the information is always up-to-date, being coherent between the server's repository and the local database of the app's instance.

The platform integrates a Web app directed to the health professional, which works as a complement to the mHealth app. It is the main interface for the health professional since it can present more detailed information about her/his patients. The Web app integrates a more complete and interactive dashboard than the mobile interface, allowing better monitoring and remote support of the therapy outside the clinic context. An important feature of this Web app is an interface in which the health professional adds new therapeutic exercises to the platform and creates programs based on them towards her/his patients. Figure 3 illustrates the main components of the platform.

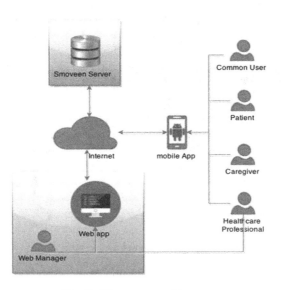

**Fig. 3.** The system architecture.

# 4   User Study

The ONParkinson R&D team has being following an iterative design process. Therefore, until now, first the concept and then the mobile app prototype have been tested by different users at different times and for different purposes. A preliminary user study was conducted to validate the ONParkinson's concept and the potential needs of the triad users [6]. Results highlighted the importance of implementing an mHealth based platform to support a remote healthcare assistance, with most of participants identifying it as "extremely relevant" [6].

A first test round with triad users started as soon as the team got a functional prototype. We carried out user tests with the ONParkinson mobile prototype in order to evaluate the acceptance of the modules and functionalities included in this first version, besides the overall usability of the application. This study was important to assess if the mHealth solution was being developed in the intended direction.

## 4.1   Design

The users testing conducted in this study comprised accomplishing tasks and post-test questionnaires. The ONParkinson team divided the tests in two parts, measuring the overall usability quality of the app using the European Portuguese version of the System Usability Scale (SUS) [13], as well the user satisfaction regarding the main modules (both parts using a seven-point Likert-type scale, which ranged from strongly disagree (1) to strongly agree (7)).

The user tests were conducted with a total of 14 participants from the Portuguese Parkinson Disease Association (literally Associação Portuguesa de Doentes de Parkinson - APDPk), including 5 people with PD (2 female; average age of 64 ± 5.92), 5 carers (1 female; average age of 66 ± 15.34), and 4 health professionals (2 female; 3 physiotherapists and 1 speech therapist). From these set groups, people with PD were the participants' group that reported a lower use of smartphones in their daily life (3 of the 5). On the other hand, only one carer did not use, and all health professionals were smartphones users. Figure 4 illustrates how the ONParkinson team conducted the usability tests with participants at the Association. A cared supervision was needed.

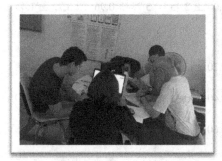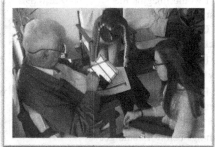

**Fig. 4.** Usability tests process: ONParkinson team with participants (patients and carers).

## 4.2   Findings

According to the first part of the tests, based on SUS, the ONParkinson app has proven to be easy to use (mean = 6.65; SD = .53) and with few inconsistencies in the system (mean = 1.28; SD = .61). Most of the SUS statements were classified equally within the triad end-users. However, differences seemed to be found in the possibility of using the app frequently. People with PD answered positively (mean = 5.6; SD = .89), but lower than their carers (mean = 6.4; SD = .89) and health professionals (mean = 6.75; SD = .50), which may indicate the importance of a deeper understanding of their motivations and expectations for its use, and more specifically, in the context of the triad's interaction using the app. Table 1 shows the complete results obtained from the SUS questionnaire, which demonstrate that the usability evaluation was overall very positive.

**Table 1.**  Results of the user tests' first part based on SUS.

| Statements | People with PD | Carers | Health professionals | Total |
|---|---|---|---|---|
| S1: I think that I would like to use ONParkinson frequently | 5,60 ± 0,89 | 6,40 ± 0,89 | 6,75 ± 0,50 | 6,25 ± 0,76 |
| S2: I found ONParkinson unnecessarily complex | 2,40 ± 1,52 | 3,20 ± 3,03 | 2,50 ± 1,00 | 2,70 ± 1,85 |
| S3: I thought ONParkinson was easy to use | 6,60 ± 0,55 | 6,60 ± 0,55 | 6,75 ± 0,50 | 6,65 ± 0,53 |
| S4: I think that I would need the support of a technical person to be able to use ONParkinson | 3,60 ± 2,30 | 2,20 ± 1,30 | 2,50 ± 2,38 | 2,77 ± 1,99 |
| S5: I found the various functions in ONParkinson were well integrated | 6,40 ± 0,55 | 6,20 ± 1,30 | 6,25 ± 0,50 | 6,28 ± 0,78 |
| S6: I thought there was too much inconsistency in ONParkinson | 1,40 ± 0,89 | 1,20 ± 0,45 | 1,25 ± 0,50 | 1,28 ± 0,61 |
| S7: I would imagine that most people would learn to use ONParkinson very quickly | 6,40 ± 0,89 | 5,00 ± 2,45 | 5,75 ± 0,96 | 5,72 ± 1,43 |
| S8: I found ONParkinson very cumbersome to use | 1,40 ± 0,55 | 2,20 ± 2,68 | 1,00 ± 0,00 | 1,53 ± 1,08 |
| S9: I felt very confident using ONParkinson | 5,80 ± 1,30 | 6,40 ± 0,89 | 6,25 ± 0,50 | 6,15 ± 0,90 |
| S10: I needed to learn a lot of things before I could get going with ONParkinson | 2,20 ± 2,17 | 1,60 ± 1,34 | 1,50 ± 0,58 | 1,77 ± 1,36 |

For a first prototype, the SUS score was very high with a value of 84.4 out of 100, meaning the ONParkinson mobile app obtains an A grade, which is the best possible. This grade also indicates that participants are more likely to be recommending the product to another potential end-user. These positive results, somewhat above the expectations, may be related to the way in which the participants' selection took place at APDPk. People who wanted to participate are possibly those who are most interested and predisposed to use new technologies and solutions based on mobile devices. Moreover, during the tests, several participants reported they wanted very much that the prototype would reach the final version in order to be able to use it on a daily basis. However, despite the very positive global results, the SUS scores of two participants were weaker since a person with PD obtained a value of 65.0 and a carer obtained only 55.0. We were expecting to obtain some scores like these two since we were dealing with people who could present obvious limitations, whether they were due to the disease or age, whose average was over 60 years.

With regard to the second part of the tests, Table 2 shows a summary of the results about three characteristics of the "app's image" (global design, logo, and font size) and the main modules/functionalities (Information, Exercises and Calendar), which were globally perceived as being well integrated. Moreover, the first two statements received the highest scores, which illustrates how much participants really liked the concept and image that is being followed by the ONParkinson development.

**Table 2.** Results of the user tests' second part regarding user satisfaction with specific aspects.

| Statements | People with PD | Carers | Health professionals | Total |
|---|---|---|---|---|
| S1: The app has an attractive design | 6,50 ± 0,58 | 6,20 ± 0,84 | 6,50 ± 0,58 | 6,40 ± 0,67 |
| S2: The logo is suitable for the app | 7,00 ± 0,00 | 5,60 ± 1,52 | 7,00 ± 0,00 | 6,53 ± 0,51 |
| S3: Font size is appropriated | 6,50 ± 0,58 | 5,80 ± 1,30 | 6,50 ± 0,58 | 6,27 ± 0,82 |
| S4: The functionality "Information" has useful and proper information | 6,25 ± 0,50 | 6,40 ± 0,89 | 6,25 ± 0,50 | 6,30 ± 0,63 |
| S5: It was easy to create and access to the events in the "Calendar" | 6,50 ± 0,58 | 5,80 ± 1,10 | 6,50 ± 0,58 | 6,27 ± 0,75 |
| S6: The functionality "Exercises" is easy to follow | 6,75 ± 0,50 | 6,20 ± 0,45 | 6,75 ± 0,50 | 6,57 ± 0,48 |

Additionally, users contributed with qualitative feedback and recommendations for improving the experience of the app. For instance, textual descriptions on the Information module were perceived as too long for some users, mainly for people with PD and carers. Health professionals recommended an increase of the number of exercises that may be selected from the ONParkinson's repository.

## 5  Conclusions and Further Work

Based on the measured user experience, this study demonstrated that the ONParkinson development is on the right path, with a high acceptance by the potential end-users, and proposed recommendations for enhancing the usability of the app.

We will continue gathering feedback while developing the prototype, assessing each one of its modules with the end-users. As part of this ongoing process, we are selecting a group of end-users that should participate in all user tests. Improving the usability of the ONParkinson mobile app may enhance the user experience to engage mainly the patients and their carers.

**Acknowledgments.** We would like to thank the students Patricia Garcia, Daniel Costa and Natália Scerbacov for their participation in the development of the prototype and collaboration in the users testing at APDPk. We also wish to thank APDPk for providing the support needed for the testings with the potential end-users.

## References

1. World Health Organization: mHealth. New horizons for health through mobile technologies (2011). http://www.who.int/goe/publications/goe_mhealth_web.pdf. Accessed 27 Sep 2016
2. Steinhubl, M.D., Muse, E.D., Topol, E.J.: Can mobile health technologies transform health care? J. Am. Med. Assoc. **310**(22), 2395–2396 (2013)
3. Kalia, L., Lang, A.: Parkinson's disease. Lancet **386**, 896–912 (2015)
4. Dorsey, E.R., Constantinescu, R., et al.: Projected number of people with Parkinson disease in the most populous nations, 2005 through 2030. Neurology **68**, 384–386 (2007)
5. European Commission: Neurodegenerative Disorders (2015). http://ec.europa.eu/health/major_chronic_diseases/diseases/brain_neurological. Accessed 25 June 2015
6. Pereira, C., Macedo, P., Madeira, R.: Mobile integrated assistance to empower people coping with parkinson's disease. In: ASSETS 2015, pp. 409–410. ACM (2015)
7. Pan, D., Dhall, R., Lieberman, A., Petitti, D.B.: A mobile cloud-based parkinson's disease assessment system for home-based monitoring. JMIR Mhealth Uhealth **3**(1), e29 (2015)
8. Patel, S., et al.: Monitoring motor fluctuations in patients with Parkinson's disease using wearable sensors. IEEE Trans. Inf. Technol. Biomed. **13**(6), 864–873 (2009)
9. Barros, A.C., Cevada, J., Bayés, A., Alcaine, S., Mestre, B.: User-centred design of a mobile self-management solution for Parkinson's disease. In: Proceedings of 12th International Conference on Mobile and Ubiquitous Multimedia (MUM 2013), Article 23, 10 p. ACM (2013)
10. Bot, B., Suver, C., Neto, E.C., et al.: The mPower study, Parkinson disease mobile data collected using ResearchKit. Sci. Data **3**, 160011, 1–9 (2016)
11. Trend, P., Kaye, J., Gage, H., Owen, C., Wade, D.: Short-term effectiveness of intensive multidisciplinary rehabilitation for people with Parkinson's disease and their carers. Clin. Rehabil. **16**, 717–725 (2002)
12. Nunes, F., Verdezoto, N., Fitzpatrick, G., Kyng, M., Grönvall, E., Storni, C.: Self-care technologies in HCI: trends, tensions, and opportunities. ACM Trans. Comput.-Hum. Interact. **22**(6), Article 33, 45 p. (2015)
13. Martins, A., Rosa, A., Queirós, A., Silva, A., Rocha, N.: European Portuguese validation of the System Usability Scale (SUS). Procedia Comput. Sci. **67**, 293–300 (2015)

# A Process for Selecting and Validating Awe-Inducing Audio-Visual Stimuli

Alice Chirico[1(⊠)], Pietro Cipresso[2], Giuseppe Riva[1,2],
and Andrea Gaggioli[1,2]

[1] Department of Psychology, Università Cattolica del Sacro Cuore, Milan, Italy
{alice.chirico,andrea.gaggioli}@unicatt.it
[2] Applied Technology for Neuro-Psychology Lab,
Istituto Auxologico Italiano, Milan, Italy
{p.cipresso,a.gaggioli}@auxologico.it

**Abstract.** Awe is a complex emotion that influences positively individuals' wellbeing both at a physical and at a psychological level. Eliciting awe in a lab setting is a delicate task, and several effective techniques have been developed to pursue this goal, such as audio-video stimuli. Nevertheless, a standardized procedure to select these audio-video awe-inducing stimuli is still needed. Therefore, we validated a methodology to select and discriminate among awe-inducing stimuli. The novelty of the methodology is two-fold: (i) it allows testing whether each content elicited the target emotion, and (ii) it allows to identify the most awe-conductive videos, using both classical statistics and Bayesian analyses. Four videos displaying awe, amusement and neutral contents were shown to participants in a counterbalanced order. This procedure allowed for identifying and validating awe-inducing stimuli that can be pliably used to improve individual's wellbeing and mental health in different contexts.

**Keywords:** Awe · Wellbeing · Mood-induction · Emotions · Bayesian

## 1 Introduction

Awe is generally considered as an emotion dwelling on the extremes of fear and pleasure [1]. Therefore, recently, it received the label of "complex", due also the fact that it encompasses opposite trends both in terms of valence and appraisal. In particular, according to Keltner and Haidt [1] feeling of awe can be flavoured both by positive and negative themes (i.e., beauty, virtue, power, threat, uncanny), and it arises from two distinct patterns of appraisal, namely "perceived vastness" and "need for accommodation". In other words, two requirements need to be simultaneously satisfied for a stimulus in order to elicit awe. First, stimuli need to be perceived as vast, both at a physical (e.g., high mountains) and at a conceptual level (e.g., complex mathematical theories). Further, awe elicitors question individual's mental frames, in order to induce a need to accommodate these previous schemas in accordance to new information.

In the psychological field, awe is regarded as one of the main drivers in individuals' life, changing profoundly people's perspective towards world and themselves [2]. More

© ICST Institute for Computer Sciences, Social Informatics and Telecommunications Engineering 2018
N. Oliver et al. (Eds.): MindCare 2016/Fabulous 2016/IIoT 2015, LNICST 207, pp. 19–27, 2018.
https://doi.org/10.1007/978-3-319-74935-8_3

pragmatically, this emotion leads to medium and long-time consequences on people' psychological [3, 4] and physical wellbeing [5].

Considering the scientific and practical relevance of this emotion, how to induce awe into experimental setting, is a significant methodological challenge. Most of the available experimental studies agree on using awe-inducing videos based on different kinds of natural phenomena. Nevertheless, two needs emerged from this field. First, the identification of clearer and unambiguous awe-inducing stimuli. Further, a standardized procedure is needed to validate these stimuli, in order to classify them as awe elicitors.

In details, to date, researchers have applied a "discriminant" methodology to select awe inducing stimuli (e.g., [4]). In other words, they asked participants to what extent they felt several discrete emotions including awe, basing only on differences among these emotions (i.e., they carried out simple One-Way ANOVAR or Within ANOVA). Thus, they did not deepen the analysis of the impact of other potential intervenient emotions elicited by the same content. According to literature [6, 7], since awe is a complex emotion encompassing both positive and negative valence, there are some emotions that can be secondary elicited by awe-inducing stimuli, but other that should not be induced by such stimuli. In this regard, multiple comparisons among emotions cannot be enough to identify a pure awe-inducing stimuli, but it is also necessary to consider similarities with emotions elicited by other control conditions, such as neutral stimuli. To address this issue, we introduced a mood induction procedure designed for eliciting awe, or other complex emotions. To reach a higher sense of immersion and isolation, even in a controlled setting, we used a VR device. The main novelty of our contribution is three-fold: (i) the encoding of a standardized mood induction procedure to elicit awe and other complex emotions; (ii) the identification of two new awe-inducing stimuli; (iii) the induction of awe by means of a VR device.

To date, awe has been measured only with respect to other emotions, therefore we included a further emotional content (i.e., "amusement"; intended to elicit an emotion that was commonly used to contrast the effect of awe [6, 8, 9]), and a control condition (i.e., an emotional neutral content was selected to control for effect of other potentially intervenient emotions [6, 10]).

The validity of the proposed methodology was tested according to the following hypotheses/criteria:

1. Stimuli selected to induce awe elicit significant higher level of awe compared to amusement and neutral stimuli.
2. Stimuli selected to induce awe are statistically similar regarding the elicitation of awe.
3. Stimuli selected to induce amusement elicit significant higher level of amusement compared to awe and neutral stimuli.
4. Stimuli selected to induce awe and neutral stimuli elicit a statistically similar level of amusement.
5. Stimuli selected to induce awe and amusement stimuli elicit significantly higher levels of the target emotions compared to other emotions.

## 2  Methodology

### 2.1   Sample and Procedure

The study sample comprised 36 adults (18 men and 18 women) volunteers living in the Piedmont and Lombardy regions of Italy. Their mean age was 25,5 (S.D. = 4,1). We chose a within-design in which each participant watched each video once using a head-mounted device. The order of video presentation was counterbalanced for each subject. Participants stood up in an isolated room wearing a Samsung Gear VR, in which each video content was displayed. Each video session was followed by a rest phase, in which participants were invited to fill out a questionnaire concerning several different emotions they could have experienced during video exposure.

### 2.2   Measures and Instruments

**Self-report.** The extent to which participants experience several different emotions was assessed using a questionnaire composed of 8 items. In details, participants were required to report the extent (from 1 = not at all; to 7 = extremely) to which they felt each of these emotions: Anger; Awe; Disgust; Fear; Pride; Sadness, Amusement and Joy. This instrument was commonly used to assess awe compared to other emotions [6, 11, 12].

**Video.** According to guidelines provided by literature [3, 4, 6–9, 11, 13–16], we created ad hoc emotive contents (2 awe-inducing stimuli; 1 amusement-inducing stimulus; 1 neutral stimulus) by using Shotcut video editing tool. Literature suggests that awe elicitors are mainly natural (i.e. usually do not include humans [11]), and they should entail a need to accommodate as well as a perception of vastness. Moreover, awe elicitors encompass both a positive and a negative valence, that is, they can convey both pleasant and unpleasant feelings. In details, since we considered discrete emotions and not general affects, fear and joy (see "self-report" section) can be interpreted as two awe sub-components, reflecting its two poles of valence. In light of these premises, we selected the two awe inducing stimuli. The first awe inducing video (A1) showed scenes of tall trees in a forest. The latter awe-inducing video (A2) was taken from the Nebelhorn Mountain ("Drohnen Flug Übers Nebelhorn"). For each awe-inspiring video we chose the nonvocal "Deep Space Awe Inspiring Music" as a background music. Amusement video (AM) is a combination of different YouTube clip-videos about jokes, and the opening theme of *Benny Hill* Show (namely, the *Yakety Sax* composed by Boots Randolph and James Q. Rich). Finally, neutral video (N) concerned a scene of hens wandering across grass. Video are displayed on a Samsun Galaxy Note 4, using Samsung Gear VR. Each video lasted 2 min.

## 3  Data Analysis

Kolomogorov-Smirnov test of normality showed that all measures were not normally distributed. Consequently, a Wilcoxon-Signed Rank test was carried out to test for significant differences among conditions. We used the Bonferroni correction for multi-comparison in paired groups, to correct p-value (i.e., p-value should be less than 0.01 to indicate a statistically significantly difference).

Moreover, to statistically grasp awe complexity, we chose to improve the stimuli validation procedure by deepening the analysis of the relationships occurring among awe, its sub-components (i.e., joy and fear as discrete emotions related to awe), and other discrete emotions that should be not related to awe (i.e., disgust, anger, pride; sadness and amusement) across the four conditions (A1, A2; AM; N). We hypothesized that awe inducing stimuli were able to induce a statistically similar level of awe (awe 1 = awe 2 regarding the level of elicited awe), and that awe stimuli and neutral stimuli elicit a statistically similar level of amusement. Moreover, we hypothesized that other emotions, which do not pertain to awe, were significantly similar across the conditions, while other emotions related to awe were not. To test this hypothesis, we carried out the paired sample T-Test Bayes Factor (BF), namely a ratio between the likelihood of the data given null-hypothesis and the one given the alternative one [17–20]. We carried out all analyses using JASP. In this study we chose BF to compare repeated measurements under the hypothesis of similarity among them. The use of BF allowed us to states if a model in which similarity is considered can be better than a model where differences are taken in to account. BF, provided the likelihood ratio of this comparison.

## 4   Results

Result were presented in relation to the experimental hypotheses.

**H1:** Awe inducing stimuli induce a significant higher level of awe compared to amusement and neutral stimuli.

A Wilcoxon-Signed Rank test indicated that A1 and A2 induced the highest levels of awe compared to AM (A1 vs. AM: $Z = -4.100$; $p < 0.001$; A2 vs. AM: $Z = -3.999$; $p < 0.001$) and N conditions (A1 vs. N: $Z = -4.840$; $p < 0.001$; A2 vs. N: $Z = -4.861$; $p < 0.001$) (see Table 1 for descriptive statistics). At the same time, AM and N did not induce a significantly different level of awe ($Z = -2.337$; $p = 0.02$). Finally, the Wilcoxon-Signed Rank test indicated also that A1 video did not induce a statistically significantly different level of awe compared to A2 video. We deepened this result by carrying out the paired sample T-Test Bayes Factor (BF).

**H2:** Awe inducing stimuli are statistically similar regarding the elicitation of awe.

**Table 1.** The table shows the correspondence between each video content and the respective label employed in this study.

| Stimuli | Label | Content |
|---|---|---|
| Awe inducing stimulus | A1 | Mountain |
| Awe inducing stimulus | A2 | Tall trees |
| Amusement inducing stimulus | AM | Collection of sketches |
| Neutral inducing stimulus | N | Hens wandering |

To test that both A1 and A2 video elicited a statistically similar level of awe, we computed Bayes Factors to show an evidence for similar levels of awe across the two Awe conditions over the alternative model of differences in these repeated measures. Results showed a substantial effect[1] for the two conditions A1 and A2 (BF01 = 4.345; err. = 1.410e−8). In other words, A1 and A2 elicited statistically significantly similar levels of awe. H0 was not rejected (Fig. 1).

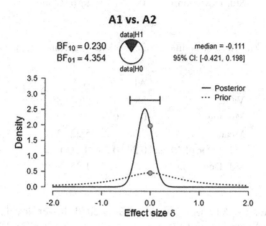

**Fig. 1.** Bayesian graph of A1 vs. A2 conditions with respect to awe measure.

**H3:** Amusement stimulus elicited a significant higher level of amusement compared to awe and neutral stimuli.
Wilcoxon-Signed Rank test showed that AM induced the highest level of amusement compared to the A1 video (Z = −4.879; p < 0.001), to A2 (Z = −4.914; p < 0.001), and to the Neutral condition (Z = −5.193; p < 0.001) (see Table 2. for descriptive statistics). AM was statistically significantly higher in AM condition relative to the Neutral (Z = −3.463; p = 0.001). A1 (Z = −3.463; p = 0.01) and A2 (Z = −1.906; p = 0.057) did not induce statistically significantly higher levels of amusement relative to the Neutral condition. As above, this last result was deepened computing the paired sample T-Test Bayes Factor (BF) (Table 3).

**H4:** Awe stimuli and neutral stimuli elicited a statistically similar level of amusement. In order to test that A1, A2 and Neutral stimuli elicited statistically similar levels of amusement, we calculated Bayes Factors, as we did for testing H2. Again, results showed a substantial effect for the condition A2 (BF01 = 3.447; err = 8.406e−9), but an anecdotal effect for A1 (BF01 = 1.473; err. = 3.288e−9). In other words, A2 did not significantly differ from Neutral regarding the level of

---

[1] Evidence in favor of the model of interest (similarity of measures) is considered anecdotal (1 &lt; BF &lt; 2.5) or substantial (2.5 &lt; BF &lt; 10). Comparing the relative predictive success of one model on another, if the BF was substantial the two measures were statistically similar relative to the hypothesis that are different. If BF < 1, it can be considered as an evidence supporting the differences instead of similarities.

**Table 2.** Descriptive statistics. Conditions are ranked according to their mean level of awe.

|                     | A1   | A2   | AM   | N    |
|---------------------|------|------|------|------|
| Valid               | 36   | 36   | 36   | 36   |
| Missing             | 0    | 0    | 0    | 0    |
| Mean                | 4.03 | 4.25 | 2.25 | 1.61 |
| Std. Error of Mean  | 0.22 | 0.29 | 0.26 | 0.15 |
| Std. Deviation      | 1.32 | 1.73 | 1.56 | 0.90 |

**Table 3.** Descriptive statistics. Conditions are ranked according to their mean level of amusement.

|                     | A1   | A2   | AM   | N    |
|---------------------|------|------|------|------|
| Valid               | 36   | 36   | 36   | 36   |
| Missing             | 0    | 0    | 0    | 0    |
| Mean                | 2.56 | 2.22 | 5.22 | 2.08 |
| Std. Error of Mean  | 0.24 | 0.26 | 0.21 | 0.23 |
| Std. Deviation      | 1.42 | 1.55 | 1.25 | 1.40 |

amusement, whereas A1 did. Indeed, A2 elicited lower levels of amusement compared to the A1 condition (A1 mean = 2.556; S.D. = 1.423; A2 mean = 2.222; S.D. = 1.551) but significantly more similar to the Neutral condition (Fig. 2).

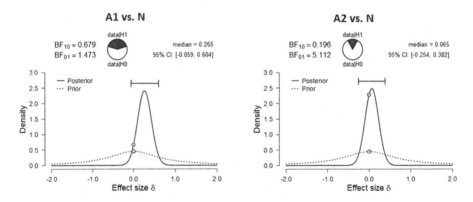

**Fig. 2.** Bayesian graph of A1 and A2 vs. N conditions considering amusement measure.

**H5:** Awe and amusement stimuli elicited significantly higher levels of the target emotions compared to other emotions. A Friedman test indicated that there were no differences in anger, pride, or sadness across conditions. Moreover, participants perceived a significantly higher level of disgust only in the Neutral condition compared to the A1 ($Z = -2.648$; $p = 0.008$). A1 and A2 elicited significantly similar levels of fear (BF01 = 4.966; err. = 1.824e−8). Further, A1 and A2 elicited the highest level of fear compared to other conditions. In details, A2 elicited a statistically significantly higher level of fear with respect to AM condition ($Z = -2.626$; $p = 0.009$). Finally, A1 and A2 elicited a significantly similar level of joy (BF01 = 5.294; err. = 2.052e−8). Further, compared to the Neutral stimulus, A1 ($Z = -4.356$; $p < 0.001$), A2 ($Z = -4.116$; $p < 0.001$) and AM elicited a significantly higher level of joy ($Z = -3.492$; $p < 0.001$). However, the levels of these secondary emotions were lower than target emotions for A1, A2 and AM.

## 5   Discussion and Conclusion

Results showed that the videos selected to induce awe and displayed by means of a VR device elicited significantly higher levels of awe compared to amusement and neutral ones. The same happened for amusement. AM video elicited the highest levels of amusement with respect to the A1, A2 video, and to the Neutral one. More interestingly, videos elicited also other secondary emotions that, however, were pertinent to the essence of awe. For example, fear belongs to the domain of awe, therefore, the fact that A1 and A2 elicited significantly similar high levels of fear is in line with literature. Nevertheless, only A2 video, which depicted scenes of tall trees, induced a level of fear significantly higher compared to AM contrast condition. At the same time, A2 elicited also a significantly higher level of Joy compared to the Neutral control condition. This suggested that A2 video resulted as a perfect interplay between positive (i.e., joy) and negative (i.e., fear) valences. In other words, since awe is a complex emotion encompassing both positive and negative valence, both A1 and A2 stimuli emerged as the closest to this definition, even A2 emerged as slightly better. Other emotions, which were unrelated to awe or amusement, did not significantly vary across conditions. Bayesian analyses combined with classic statistics help us control for every intervenient effect of other emotions, in order to clearly control for each secondary emotion potentially elicited by awe stimuli, and to identify the most awe-conductive stimulus (see Fig. 3 below for a summary of this validation procedure).

In other words, these preliminary data provided a support for the use of this new mood validation procedure, and allowed to identify two new awe-conductive stimuli. Further it provided a preliminary support for the use of video displayed on a VR device to induce awe. Finally, this procedure showed also which of these videos emerged as the most awe-conductive one (i.e., A2 video). This procedure can be implemented in different ways. First, it can be easily reproduced and applied to identify a suitable set of awe-inducing stimuli for several different contexts. This is relevant not only for research purposes, but also in clinical field, for improving individuals' wellbeing, and also for prevention. Indeed, it has been demonstrated that dispositional awe was associated with lower levels of proinflammatory cytokines, involved in the onset and development of several chronic diseases. In details, as regard to the heath context, our procedure allows for structuring ad hoc awe-training to improve physical and mental health, using not invasive, low cost standardized validated stimuli. Moreover, this procedure can be extended also to other complex emotions, such as nostalgia, maybe testing whether it is more effective than traditional mood induction techniques. For example, a 2D videos

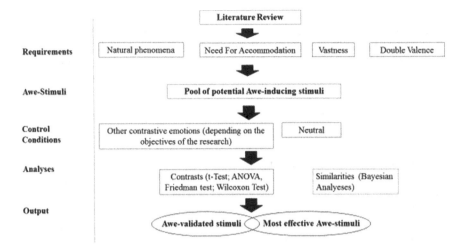

**Fig. 3.** A diagram illustrating the phases to implement this new methodology for eliciting awe using videos.

showing an awe content on a laptop monitor can be compared to the same video displayed on a head-mounted immersive display. Moreover, it could be useful in deepening the analysis of the relationship between complex emotions and health, by understanding the underlying mechanisms. Indeed, according to Riva [21], new technologies can be involved also in a process of individuals' transformation, mainly in a rehabilitative context, and this study can result as the first step to address this issue empirically. This validation procedure allows to identify suitable stimuli to elicit positive complex emotions able to trigger a transformative change process [2, 22]. For example, these stimuli can support a patient in the entire process of rehabilitation, by promoting an incisive change in his/her lifestyle. Further, this procedure could be implemented by using Virtual Reality, which has already resulted as a suitable and successful methodology of mood induction [23, 24]. Finally, some limitations concern the small sample, thus it could be useful to further analyze these data separately, according to each subgroup. Finally, a possibility to improve this research could be introducing measures of psychological wellbeing [25], and coping strategies [26], as well as assessing the ongoing awe experience, through psychophysiological measures.

# References

1. Keltner, D., Haidt, J.: Approaching awe, a moral, spiritual, and aesthetic emotion. Cogn. Emot. **17**(2), 297–314 (2003)
2. Schneider, K.J.: Awakening to Awe: Personal Stories of Profound Transformation. Jason Aronson, Lanham (2009)
3. Krause, N., Hayward, R.D.: Assessing whether practical wisdom and awe of god are associated with life satisfaction. Psychol. Relig. Spirituality **7**(1), 51 (2015)
4. Rudd, M., Vohs, K.D., Aaker, J.: Awe expands people's perception of time, alters decision making, and enhances well-being. Psychol. Sci. **23**(10), 1130–1136 (2012)

5. Stellar, J.E., John-Henderson, N., Anderson, C.L., Gordon, A.M., McNeil, G.D., Keltner, D.: Positive affect and markers of inflammation: discrete positive emotions predict lower levels of inflammatory cytokines. Emotion **15**(2), 129 (2015)
6. Piff, P.K., Piff, P.K., Dietze, P., Feinberg, M., Stancato, D.M., Keltner, D.: Awe, the small self, and prosocial behavior. J. Pers. Soc. Psychol. **108**(6), 883 (2015)
7. Shiota, M.N., Keltner, D., Mossman, A.: The nature of awe: elicitors, appraisals, and effects on self-concept. Cogn. Emot. **21**(5), 944–963 (2007)
8. Valdesolo, P., Graham, J.: Awe, uncertainty, and agency detection. Psychol. Sci. **25**(3), 844 (2014)
9. Van Cappellen, P., Saroglou, V.: Awe activates religious and spiritual feelings and behavioral intentions. Psychol. Relig. Spirituality **4**(3), 223 (2012)
10. Griskevicius, V., Shiota, M.N., Neufeld, S.L.: Influence of different positive emotions on persuasion processing: a functional evolutionary approach. Emotion **10**(2), 190 (2010)
11. Prade, C., Saroglou, V.: Awe's effects on generosity and helping. J. Positive Psychol. **11**, 1–9 (2016)
12. Saroglou, V., Buxant, C., Tilquin, J.: Positive emotions as leading to religion and spirituality. J. Positive Psychol. **3**(3), 165–173 (2008)
13. Bonner, E.: Exploring dispositional awe and its relationship with spiritual intelligence: measuring dispositional awe as a multidimensional construct. Northcentral University (2015)
14. Schurtz, D.R., Blincoe, S., Smith, R.H., Powell, C.A., Combs, D.J., Kim, S.H.: Exploring the social aspects of goose bumps and their role in awe and envy. Motiv. Emot. **36**(2), 205–217 (2012)
15. Sundararajan, L.: Religious awe: potential contributions of negative theology to psychology, "positive" or otherwise. J. Theor. Philos. Psychol. **22**(2), 174 (2002)
16. Yaden, D.B., et al.: The overview effect: awe and self-transcendent experience in space flight. Psychol. Conscious. Theory Res. Pract. **3**(1), 1–11 (2016)
17. Liang, F., Paulo, R., Molina, G., Clyde, M.A., Berger, J.O.: Mixtures of g priors for Bayesian variable selection. J. Am. Stat. Assoc. **103**(481), 410–423 (2012)
18. Masson, M.E.: A tutorial on a practical Bayesian alternative to null-hypothesis significance testing. Behav. Res. Methods **43**(3), 679–690 (2011)
19. Nuzzo, R.: Statistical errors. Nature **506**(7487), 150–152 (2014)
20. Rouder, J.N.: Optional stopping: no problem for Bayesians. J. Probl. Solving **21**(2), 301–308 (2014)
21. Riva, G., Villani, D., Cipresso, P., Repetto, C., Triberti, S., Di Lernia, D., Chirico, A., Serino, A., Gaggioli, A.: Positive and transformative technologies for active ageing. Stud. Health Technol. Inform. **220**, 308–315 (2016)
22. Chirico, A., Yaden, D., Riva, G., Gaggioli, A.: The potential of virtual reality for the investigation of awe. Front. Psychol. **7**(1766) (2016). https://doi.org/10.3389/fpsyg.2016.01766
23. Felnhofer, A., Kothgassner, O.D., Schmidt, M., Heinzle, A.-K., Beutl, L., Hlavacs, H., Kryspin-Exner, I.: Is virtual reality emotionally arousing? Investigating five emotion inducing virtual park scenarios. Int. J. Hum. Comput. Stud. **82**, 48–56 (2015)
24. Gorini, A., Capideville, C.S., De Leo, G., Mantovani, F., Riva, G.: The role of immersion and narrative in mediated presence: the virtual hospital experience. Cyberpsychol. Behav. Soc. Network. **14**(3), 99–105 (2011)
25. Dupuy, H.: The Psychological General Well-Being (PGWB) inventory. In: Wenger, N. (ed.) Assessment of Quality of Life in Clinical Trials of Cardiovascular Therapies, pp. 170–183. Le Jacq Publications, New York (1984)
26. Carver, C.S., Scheier, M.F., Weintraub, J.J.: Assessing coping strategies: a theoretically based approach. J. Pers. Soc. Psychol. **56**, 267–283 (1989)

# A Play Therapy Based Full-Body Interaction Intervention Tool for Children with Autism

Joan Mora-Guiard[✉] [ID], Ciera Crowell, and Narcis Pares

University Pompeu Fabra, Carrer Roc Boronat 138, 08018 Barcelona, Spain
{joan.mora, ciera.crowell, narcis.pares}@upf.edu

**Abstract.** Autism Spectrum Disorders (ASD) are characterized by social and communication difficulties, which can result in challenges forming relationships with peers and taking part in imaginative play. Play Therapy creates recreational spaces where children can learn social skills in an exploratory and creative manner. As children with ASD have a unique affinity towards computer based systems, play therapy approaches using Information and Communication Technologies (ICT) have proved useful in maintaining player motivation and engagement. In this article we will present an intervention tool inspired by play therapy that we have designed using full-body interaction technology, which has been successful in fostering social behaviors in children with ASD.

**Keywords:** Autism · ASD · Play therapy · Full-body interaction

## 1 Introduction

As children, play provides a safe space for developing the imagination and exploring creative narratives. According to Wieder et al. [66], play is the most important part of childhood, where children can share and explore thoughts and feelings. It is a time when children can distance themselves from real life enough to think in abstract terms, assigning symbolic meanings to everyday items. In the case of children with developmental disorders like Autism Spectrum Disorders (ASD), the imaginative world can expand regardless of the boundaries placed on physical and sensory means. In fact, research has shown the potential of play-based therapies in the development of social and communication behaviors in children with ASD [18].

Play can be built within or around the boundaries of game rules, or objects, while retaining a certain degree of freedom for creative construction [17]. The degree of interpretation given to players is dictated by whether the play arrangement is open-ended or goal oriented. Open ended play refrains from strict structural elements, and allows children to create their own rules for play [10]. For example, when given a plastic ball, children will begin to propose and negotiate play dynamics, all the while exploring the properties of the play object. In this process, creativity is drawn from each player's subjective frame of reference, mixing them with the experience and suggestions of other players [51].

In an experiment by Dewey et al. [25], it was found that rule based games were considered the most fun, and yielded the most complex interactions. However, when

© ICST Institute for Computer Sciences, Social Informatics and Telecommunications Engineering 2018
N. Oliver et al. (Eds.): MindCare 2016/Fabulous 2016/IIoT 2015, LNICST 207, pp. 28–40, 2018.
https://doi.org/10.1007/978-3-319-74935-8_4

children were given glowing play balls in an experiment by Bekker et al. [10], it was observed that children liked playing more in free-play sessions than in game sessions with pre-defined goals.

In order to create an enjoyable, and more importantly, engaging, play experience, certain factors must be taken into account. In the realm of computer game development, there must exist a balance between sense of control, the chance to create strategies, and the search for new information [53]. Maintaining player engagement means the game play must also uphold a certain degree of challenge. These challenges are supported by clear goals and attainable goals which the player must work towards during the course of play [52]. When the challenge of a game is met with feelings of enjoyment, the player enters the moment of "flow" [21], which is considered a highly concentrated and fulfilling state [33]. Moreover, players can maintain motivation through feedback such as positive reinforcements, which can be a valuable tool in the process of developing new skills for children with developmental disorders such as ASD [47].

## 1.1 Autism Spectrum Disorder

Autism Spectrum Disorders are a collection of neurodevelopmental conditions which impact an individual's propensity for social communication and social interaction [6]. Although people with ASD show a wide range of intellectual and motor capabilities [63], there are a few characteristics which are particularly common among diagnosed individuals. These include inhibitions in social communication and restricted, repetitive behaviors.

## 1.2 Social Difficulties with ASD

The pervasive deficits in social abilities among individuals with ASD frequently result in challenges in developing, maintaining, and understanding relationships with others. Individuals with ASD may show difficulties in social-emotional reciprocity, taking part in imaginative play, or initiating social interactions. As a result, children with ASD typically engage in a higher frequency of solitary, nonsocial play [44] and may have a higher incidence of social fragmentation in friendship and classroom circles [3].

Along with conversation, individuals with ASD also have difficulties understanding non-verbal language, which can lead to misinterpretations of unspoken social norms and expectations [24] or failure to detect contextual meanings of words [35]. Individuals with ASD also find seeking involvement and acceptance difficult, resulting in problems carrying out collaborative tasks [65].

Research has shown that early intervention in children with high-functioning ASD leads to better progress reports [67], thus increasing the potential for an improved quality of life.

## 1.3 Play Therapy

Play therapy is a set of play-based interventions, where a therapist builds communication with patients through driving play activities towards patients' interests. It is commonly used as an intervention for the development of social and communication skills. Research evidences the efficacy of play-based therapy [15] and its specific benefits for the acquisition of social and communication skills [18]. Thus, play has potential as intervention given its structured nature upon which participants can build new needs and interactions.

Children with ASD tend to show uncommon behaviors in imaginative and symbolic play when interacting with objects. Their approach to toys tends to be an exploration through taste and touch [60], becoming intimate and close to the objects. Nonetheless, playing is crucial in children with ASD as, although they might approach objects differently than neurotypically developing children, they can express themselves naturally through play. The Developmental, Individual-Difference, Relationship-Based (DIR) model, known as Floortime [66] is one form of child-led play therapy which consists of six milestones, including relationship building and complex communication. Bratton et al. found that humanistic non-directed play therapies produce significantly larger effects than non-humanistic directive therapies [15]. Non-directed interventions for children with ASD have been proven to be effective therapy [40]. The project we present in this article seeks for a humanistic non-directed intervention, as the system was designed to help children recognize their creativity and freedom by letting them play without enforcing any specific play style.

One of the most successful and known research projects on play-based therapy for children with ASD is by Legoff [42]. Legoff used LEGO brick sets as a tool for mediating communication between groups of children with high functioning ASD. During experimental sessions each child had a specific role in the building process, thus all children in each group were forced to cooperate and collaborate to achieve the final goal. The results showed an improvement in the acquisition of social abilities, specifically initialization of peer contact.

## 2   State of the Art

In an attempt to provide engaging and dynamic interventions, many research efforts have utilized Information and Communication Technologies (ICT) to create play and learning experiences for children with ASD [34]. Furthermore, it has been shown that children with ASD have a special interest in computerized learning [12], possibly due to the linear and systematic nature of most computer programs [16]. This clear structure can reduce anxiety for individuals with ASD, as they usually show increased responsiveness to stimuli when events are predictable [29]. Also, with ICT, change can be introduced and mediated in a discrete manner [2].

Various kinds of ICT have been shown to be effective for use in treatment and learning. Projects which use computer graphics displays have been recommended with ASD for the use of visually cued instructions. Examples include hand held devices for aiding communication [49], tangible user interfaces (TUI) for learning social communication skills [48], and multi-touch tabletops for teaching group collaboration [8]. Children with ASD have also shown positive responses to working with robots for practicing imitation and joint attention [28].

## 2.1 Virtual Reality Intervention for Autism

Virtual reality is a type of ICT which uses real time virtual displays which can represent real or imaginary events and environments [54]. These systems can provide a safe training environment to practice social behaviors, without the distraction of external stimuli [1]. VR approaches have proven beneficial for individuals with ASD in planning, problem solving, and management of behavior [64]. Examples of virtual reality interventions include head mounted displays for simulating real life situations [61], and virtual environments for social skills training [55].

## 2.2 For Socialization

Projects for children with ASD have successfully used a variety of virtual reality approaches to teach social skills. Social training can take place through simulation of everyday places, such as being in a restaurant [62], a birthday party [41], or a bus [55]. Virtual reality and multimedia approaches can also represent magical or imaginary situations to appeal to children's interests, such as a troll forest [68], an enchanted world [50], or an alien planet [32, 45]. Social skills training can also create a collaborative environment, where multiple users work together. Examples of collaborative ICT projects include solving a puzzle with a partner [8] and creating an apple orchard narrative [32]. The use of virtual agents as digital peers can be a valuable tool for teaching collaboration and to reduce avoidance mechanisms [2].

# 3 Full-Body Interaction

Full-body interactive technologies pose a unique stance to the interactive technologies paradigm, placing the body as the center of interaction [50]. These interactive technologies are operated by the natural gestures used in daily life for expression and communication, through the movements of the body and under-standing oneself as an active participant in relation to the surrounding physical and virtual space.

Virtual environments allow the user to have control over senses, movement, and communication in the virtual setting [20]. As individuals with ASD commonly have difficulties with motor skills [43], full-body virtual environments allow a freedom of movement beyond the traditional mouse and screen setup [19]. Full-body technologies in particular have been seen to assist in learning [5, 39]. Also, collocated full-body experiences allow for face-to-face collaboration withother users, which has been seen to foster social behavior [50]. This research shows that full-body interaction systems hold potential as intervention tools for individuals with social disabilities, such as autism.

The theoretical basis for full-body interaction may be understood as a dynamic relationship between cognitive processes and the subjective human experience that we construct by living and moving within the world. In fact, embodied cognition theories hold that cognition is mediated by the human body and its place within the surroundings [13]. It is this relation between body and space which defines our human condition [24], placing knowledge not as an abstract concept to be passed from one person to another, but rather a contextual construction which is influenced by our previously held perceptions and experiences. This perspective, known as situated learning, sets learning as a social activity between humans as constructors of knowledge [56]. Therefore, meaning is created as we collaboratively interact with others and the world around us [31].

In the field of Human-Computer Interaction, embodied interaction takes the human as an active participant in the particular setting [27]. This concept of embodied interaction aims for direct manipulation of the virtual environment, also by collaborative user groups [4, 26]. In addition, as emotion is seen to be connected to cognition and understanding of information [36], full body interactive environments based in embodied interaction and user states can be advantageous for learning of concepts [58]. This was shown in an experiment by Benson and Uzgaris, where babies who were allowed to crawl through an environment found hidden objects easier than babies who had been carried through [11]. This shows how first person exploration of an environment leads to mental model construction [7]. Also, the framework of Embodied Facilitation describes how the layout of material objects and space relates to group behavior [38]. This theme is important when designing play experiences, as providing feedback to physical activity can be implemented in group settings to stimulate physical play [9].

# 4 Lands of Fog

In this section we will describe Lands of Fog, a full-body interactive play environment for children with ASD. The system allows children with ASD to play collaboratively with a neurotypical partner to learn and practice social behaviors, offering strategies to help children engage in the flow of the experience while reinforcing positive social behaviors.

The system Lands of Fog was formed as part of the IN-AUTIS-TIC project, funded by the Recercaixa 2013 grant. The project was based upon the project Lightpools, an interactive art installation with the goal of fostering socialization among users [37]. In an informal setting, the Lightpools system was tested with children with ASD and found to spark social initiation behaviors. Lightpools' interactive design was adapted to form the basis of Lands of Fog, which was created as a full-body interactive environment to foster socialization and collaboration in children with ASD. As in Lightpools, Lands of Fog utilized a 6 m in diameter, circular floor projected setting, which was considered large enoughto give each child their personal space for exploration but also small enough to encourage serendipitous encounters and meetings. The circular format was created to prevent potential isolation of children in corners and also naturally guide participants back to the middle of the physical and virtual environment.

For the design of the Lands of Fog, we conducted 5 participatory design sessions with children with ASD. Children directly defined the design of the game by contributing ideas for content and interactions. This practice falls in line with participatory design research which shows that when designing systems for individuals with special needs, is important to include their unique perspectives [30].

## 4.1   Design

In the gaming system, the virtual world is covered by a dense layer of virtual fog, which the users can partially open to reveal part of the world which lies below as they wander through the virtual scenario. The fog motivated users to adopt an active attitude towards the game by limiting viewpoints. This is referred to as a "peephole", a design strategy which Dalsgaard and Dindler suggested to promote exploration [22]. Moreover, limiting the viewing content was meant to help users focus on relevant information while exploring, as only one part of the virtual environment could be seen at a time.

Users carry a glowing butterfly net as a handheld device which works a cognitive offloader to channel the users attention into the play setting. Swarms of fireflies wander around the virtual environment, which can be caught with the butterfly net. Once caught, fireflies change their color to match their captor's net. Users understand easily the extent of their control in the system by moving around the butterfly net, and can create strategies for hunting insects, which helps children to get into the flow of the experience.

After users hunt a certain amount of fireflies, these insects will transform into a magical creature which follows the user (see Fig. 1). Each creature was designed by children with ASD in the aforementioned participatory design sessions. These creatures open a new level of interaction richness with the experience. This progression, from hunting fireflies to controlling a creature, was designed to offer the children an initial simple-to-grasp mechanic (i.e. hunting fireflies) that would foster their engagement while getting acquainted with the system. Davis et al. suggested that it was a good practice to first design features which would be easily understood by children with ASD, while novel and richer elements can be gradually introduced later on [23].

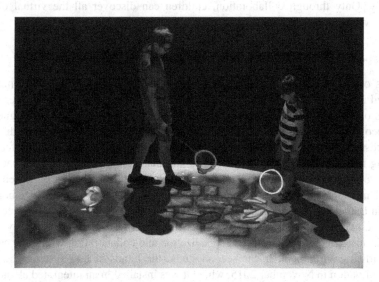

**Fig. 1.** Two players exploring the virtual environment in Lands of Fog.

If users adopt a passive attitude while playing, their creatures will try to call for their attention using positive feedback such as waving to their owner. All creature behaviors were implemented to engage users. Another example is when users are passive for a long time the creatures will try to get closer to the other user's creature. This mechanic was devised for sparking socialization behaviors between users during play.

When creatures come close, they perform a greeting action towards the other creature. We designed this so creatures would be models of social behaviors for the players. If the two users get even closer, the creatures will merge and create new creatures, which take the place of the old ones. Thus, children find that they have to collaborate if they want to discover all the creatures. If users just keep hunting fireflies, their creature will change its external appearance up to four times. The discovery of new creatures was designed as a positive reinforcement for collaboration to engage users and keep their motivation.

Apart from the creatures, the world scenario in which the users play is also populated by virtual elements which the users can interact with. As the creatures, all the virtual elements were designed during participatory design sessions. These virtual objects spark the interest of users, who share their discoveries with their partner and proceed to explore the world together. If a user approaches the virtual elements, their creature will point towards the element and make an exclamatory remark. This way the creature tries to communicate to the child that the element might be a point of interest. Again, these behaviors were devised to encourage the user to explore, and also to promote an inquisitive attitude that would foster socialization between users.

The virtual elements can only be activated when both users bring their creatures close to the element at the same time. If both creatures are close to an object, they will interact with it. The object will respond with an animation, as a positive reinforcement to collaboration, and then will disappear. Meanwhile the creatures will celebrate their discovery. Only through collaboration, children can discover all the virtual objects form the virtual world.

### 4.2 Experimental Evaluation

A series of experimental trials were carried out in Barcelona during the summer of 2015 and in London during fall of 2015. The sample included children between 10 to 15 years old with an ASD diagnosis by ADOS Model 3 diagnostic tool, designed for young people with verbal fluency. These selection criteria were chosen to include youth with autism who possessed adequate capabilities to explore the game's features, including moving freely within the scenario and conversing verbally with a partner.

We conducted two studies to evaluate the system. The first study, based on a repeated measures design with randomized couples, was in a controlled laboratory setting in Barcelona, where during the course of one month each child participated in 3 playing sessions of 15 min. The goal of this study was to evaluate the efficacy of the system in fostering user engagement, socialization and collaboration within the context of the virtual environment. In the second study, the Lands of Fog system was transported to London in November 2015, where it was installed in an integrated elementary school with a Special Educational Needs program. Over the course of one week, 20 children with ASD played in the system. An experimental protocol was defined by the researchers along with psychologists and school personnel, and it was decided that each child would play for 15 min with a typically developed classmate.

For evaluating the system we had three different data gathering methods. In Barcelona, questionnaires were administered to parents before and after each session to evaluate children's response to the experience. In London, after each session, children were interviewed, with a different questionnaires, about their experience and how they perceived their partner. The goal of these trials was to evaluate the efficacy of the system in an integrated school setting. The second method was based on video recording the sessions and subsequent coding of these with a video coding scheme designed alongside the psychologist. The last data gathering method was the activity logs generated by the system to record movement and playing data.

## 4.3 Experimental Results

The system was evaluated based upon its ability to motivate children with ASD to engage in playful social and collaborative behaviors with their partner. In the laboratory setting, we saw that the number of seconds remaining still decreased significantly from the first to the second session ($Z = -2.191$, $p = .029$) and from the first to the third session ($Z = -2.293$, $p = .022$). The number of collaborative interactions such as manipulating virtual elements increased significantly through the sessions (ANOVA: $F(2, 9) = 22.9$, $p < .05$) (Table 1). In Barcelona experimental setting, post-session questionnaires revealed that the activity level of the children was rated significantly higher by parents through the sessions (ANOVA: $F(2, 9) = 9.559$, $p < .05$) (Table 2). This marked increase in activity supports that the virtual environment motivated children to explore and play. Barcelona post-session questionnaires also revealed an increase in flexibility in the children with ASD through the playful experience with a significantly increase from the first to the second session ($Z = -2,414$, $p = .016$) and from the first to the third session ($Z = -2,060$, $p = .039$). As individuals with ASD have a tendency to adopt repetitive patterns of behavior, this change in flexibility demonstrates that the game fostered a willingness to embrace the playful acts of exploring, sharing and adopting collaborative behaviors. Multimodal data analysis revealed that in London experiments a 95% of children with ASD felt more comfortable interacting with their partner in the game setting than in physical education, and a 65% of typically developing children reported an increased willingness to get to know better their ASD playing partners.

**Table 1.** Virtual elements manipulated

| Source | N | M | SD |
|--------|---|---|-----|
| Session 1 | 10 | 4.5 | 4.2 |
| Session 2 | 10 | 16.1 | 9.2 |
| Session 3 | 10 | 23.5 | 6.6 |

**Table 2.** Activity level

| Source | N | M | SD |
|--------|---|---|-----|
| Session 1 | 10 | 4.1 | 3.14 |
| Session 2 | 10 | 5.1 | 3.48 |
| Session 3 | 10 | 4.8 | 3.59 |

We observed significant increases in social initiations and responses from the first to the third session in Barcelona experiments ($Z = -2,807$, $p = .005$) and from the second to the third session ($Z = -2,040$, $p = .041$). This means that, in the context of the playful experience, children with ASD were successful in engaging in social communication with their partner. In addition, 95% of children with ASD reported that they preferred playing with their partner in the game than in physical education class.

## 5  Discussion

By using child-led play as a model for gameplay, our aim was not to lead the children through a set of pre-defined objectives, but rather to bring out their own creative and exploratory nature as they work together with a partner to build their own understanding of the environment. Through this experience, we aimed for a non-directed spontaneous form of interaction, the same as might be found while playing on the playground or other peer-to-peer play settings. Results show that Lands of Fog was successful on motivating users to engage in collaborative play within the system, while also fostering social behaviors between players. Moreover, parent, professional and user feedback through questionnaires shows that the game was well received.

Basing the design of our intervention tool on play therapy allowed us the develop a system which could be effectively used to help children with ASD to learn and practice social and collaborative behaviors. The strategies designed for the game successfully helped children with ASD to get acquainted with the system and the control. The initial mechanics helped children to get into the flow of the experience and quickly adopt social behaviors in order to collaborate and discover the different positive rewards.

It is important to note that, although children showed increases in positive social behaviors and collaboration during the course of playing the game, these results have not been tested for generalization into other areas of their daily life.

As the longest duration of testing was over three sessions, we cannot expect that the sessions had a large impact on the neurodevelopmental condition and habits that have been formed over the course of their lives. In observing that the children were motivated to engage in the collaborative play activity, we are encouraged to see that playing with a partner can be a positive experience for these children to foster socialization. Further research must include multi-modal data collection which can help determine to what extent the children are comfortable in the collaborative play setting when interacting with their partner, and how these experiences can be built to accommodate the special tendencies that individuals with autism have regarding social interaction.

In the design of interfaces for children with special needs, several patterns have emerged as indicators of successful design. For example, including children has been held as an important aspect of the design process, as their interests, abilities and values differ greatly from adults [57]. This inclusion of children's voices can be done through participatory design studies [46]. Also, using common, recognizable objects (in our case, butterfly nets) is a way to create intuitive interaction [51].

For children with ASD, activity based learning with peers is preferred by children rather than direct instruction [14]. Constraints and structure in the system work to the benefit of children with ASD [32], along with task consistency and gradual introduction of new elements [23]. Finally, sensory reinforcers have been shown to motivate learning in young children with ASD [59].

Finally, future work should focus on assessing the system in more longitudinal studies where the system is integrated into a classroom or intervention program, so the system could be evaluated as an intervention tool for children with ASD.

## 6   Conclusions

This article presents a novel potential digital intervention tool for motivating social initiation and collaborative behaviors in children with ASD, which was inspired by humanistic non-directed play therapy and its design was informed by objective population through a series of participatory design sessions. Results of the two experimental studies we have done show that the full-body interaction system is successful in promoting social behaviors and collaboration during game play between users.

We believe that Lands of Fog demonstrates the potential of full-body interaction technology to design playful intervention systems for social communication therapy. This kind of systems could be deployed in special education centers and inclusive schools as intervention tools, but also as aids for social inclusion for children with ASD in playful settings with peers, as results show the system was successful on changing positively how peers perceived each other after playing with the system.

## References

1. Rizzo, A.S., Kim, G.J.: A SWOT analysis of the field of virtual reality rehabilitation and therapy. Presence **14**, 119–146 (2006)
2. Alcorn, A., et al.: Social communication between virtual characters and children with autism. In: Biswas, G., Bull, S., Kay, J., Mitrovic, A. (eds.) AIED 2011. LNCS (LNAI), vol. 6738, pp. 7–14. Springer, Heidelberg (2011). https://doi.org/10.1007/978-3-642-21869-9_4
3. Anderson, A., Locke, J., Kretzmann, M., Kasari, C., AIR-B Network: Social network analysis of children with autism spectrum disorder: predictors of fragmentation and connectivity in elementary school classrooms. Autism **20**, 700–709 (2015)
4. Antle, A.N.: Research opportunities: embodied child computer interaction. Int. J. Child-Computer Interact. **1**(1), 30–36 (2013)
5. Antle, A.N., Corness, G., Droumeva, M.: What the body knows: exploring the benefits of embodied metaphors in hybrid physical digital environments. Interact. Comput. **21**(1–2), 66–75 (2009)
6. American Psychiatric Association: Diagnostic and Statistical Manual of Mental Disorders, 5th edn. Washington, DC (2013)
7. Bartoli, L., Corradi, C., Garzotto, F., Valoriani, M.: Exploring motion-based touchless games for autistic children's learning. In: Proceedings of the 12th International Conference on Interaction Design and Children, IDC 2013, New York, pp. 102–111. ACM Press, June 2013
8. Battocchi, A., Pianesi, F., Tomasini, D., Zancanaro, M., Esposito, G., Venuti, P., Ben Sasson, A., Gal, E., Weiss, P.L.: Collaborative puzzle game. In: Proceedings of the ACM International Conference on Interactive Tabletops and Surfaces, ITS 2009, New York, p. 197. ACM Press, November 2009
9. Bekker, T., Sturm, J.: Stimulating physical and social activity through open-ended play. In: Proceedings of the 8th International Conference on Interaction Design and Children, IDC 2009, New York, p. 309. ACM Press, June 2009

10. Bekker, T., Sturm, J., Wesselink, R., Groenendaal, B., Eggen, B.: Interactive play objects and the effects of open-ended play on social interaction and fun. In: Proceedings of Advances in Computer Entertainment Technology, pp. 389–392 (2008)
11. Benson, J.B., Užgiris, I.Č.: Effect of self-initiated locomotion on infant search activity. Dev. Psychol. **21**(6), 923–931 (1985)
12. Bernard-Opitz, V., Sriram, N., Nakhoda-Sapuan, S.: Enhancing social problem solving in children with autism and normal children through computer-assisted instruction. J. Autism Dev. Disord. **31**(4), 377–384 (2001)
13. Borghi, A.M., Cimatti, F.: Embodied cognition and beyond: acting and sensing the body. Neuropsychologia **48**(3), 763–773 (2010)
14. Bottema-Beutel, K., Mullins, T.S., Harvey, M.N., Gustafson, J.R., Carter, E.W.: Avoiding the "brick wall of awkward": perspectives of youth with autism spectrum disorder on social-focused intervention practices. Autism Int. J. Res. Pract. (2015). https://doi.org/10.1177/1362361315574888
15. Bratton, S.C., Ray, D., Rhine, T., Jones, L.: The efficacy of play therapy with children: a meta-analytic review of treatment outcomes. Prof. Psychol. Res. Pract. **36**(4), 376–390 (2005)
16. Brown, J., Murray, D.: Strategies for enhancing play skills for children with autism spectrum disorder. Educ. Train. Ment. Retard. Dev. Disabil. **36**(3), 312–317 (2001)
17. Caillois, R., Barash, M.: Man, Play, and Games. University of Illinois Press, Champaign (1961)
18. Casenhiser, D.M., Shanker, S.G., Stieben, J.: Learning through interaction in children with autism: preliminary data from asocial-communication-based intervention. Autism Int. J. Res. Pract. **17**(2), 220–241 (2013)
19. Chen, W.: Multitouch tabletop technology for people with autism spectrum disorder: a review of the literature. Procedia Comput. Sci. **14**, 198–207 (2012)
20. Cobb, S., Parsons, S., Millen, L., Eastgate, R., Glover, T.: Design and development of collaborative technology for children with autism: COSPATIAL, March 2010
21. Csikszentmihalyi, M.: Creativity: Flow and the Psychology of Discovery and Invention. Harper Collins Publishers, New York (1996)
22. Dalsgaard, P., Dindler, C.: Between theory and practice. In: Proceedings of the 32nd Annual ACM Conference on Human Factors in Computing Systems, CHI 2014, New York, pp. 1635–1644. ACM Press, April 2014
23. Davis, M., Dautenhahn, K., Powell, S.D., Nehaniv, C.L.: Guidelines for researchers and practitioners designing software and software trials for children with autism. J. Assist. Technol. **4**(1), 38–48 (2010)
24. De Jaegher, H.: Embodiment and sense-making in autism. Front. Integr. Neurosci. **7**, 15 (2013)
25. Dewey, D., Lord, C., Magill, J.: Qualitative assessment of the effect of play materials in dyadic peer interactions of children with autism. Can. J. Psychol. **42**(2), 242–260 (1988)
26. Dillenbourg, P., Evans, M.: Interactive tabletops in education. Int. J. Comput. Support. Collab. Learn. **6**(4), 491–514 (2011)
27. Dourish, P.: Where the Action Is: The Foundations of Embodied Interaction. MIT Press, Cambridge (2001)
28. Duquette, A., Michaud, F., Mercier, H.: Exploring the use of a mobile robot as an imitation agent with children with low-functioning autism. Auton. Robots **24**(2), 147–157 (2007)
29. Ferrara, C., Hill, S.D.: The responsiveness of autistic children to the predictability of social and nonsocial toys. J. Autism Dev. Disord. **10**(1), 51–57 (1980)

30. Frauenberger, C., Good, J., Alcorn, A., Pain, H.: Supporting the design contributions of children with autism spectrum conditions. In: Proceedings of the 11th International Conference on Interaction Design and Children, pp. 134–143 (2012)
31. Fuchs, T., de Jaegher, H.: Enactive intersubjectivity: participatory sense-making and mutual incorporation. Phenomenol. Cogn. Sci. **8**, 465–486 (2009)
32. Giusti, L., Zancanaro, M., Gal, E., Weiss, P.L.T.: Dimensions of collaboration on a tabletop interface for children with autism spectrum disorder. In: Proceedings of the 2011 Annual Conference on Human Factors in Computing Systems, CHI 2011, New York, p. 3295. ACM Press, May 2011
33. Goh, D.H., Ang, R.P., Tan, H.C.: Strategies for designing effective psychotherapeutic gaming interventions for children and adolescents. Comput. Hum. Behav. **24**(5), 2217–2235 (2008)
34. Goldsmith, T.R., LeBlanc, L.A.: Use of technology in interventions for children with autism
35. Grynszpan, O., Martin, J.C., Nadel, J.: Multimedia interfaces for users with high functioning autism: an empirical investigation. Int. J. Hum. Comput. Stud. **66**(8), 628–639 (2008)
36. Harrison, S., Tatar, D., Sengers, P.: The three paradigms of HCI. In: CHI, San Jose, USA, pp. 1–21 (2007)
37. Hoberman, P., Pares, N., Pares, R.: El ball del fanalet or lightpools. In: Proceedings of International Conference on Virtual Systems and Multimedia, January 1999
38. Hornecker, E., Buur, J.: Getting a grip on tangible interaction. In: Proceedings of the SIGCHI Conference on Human Factors in Computing Systems, CHI 2006, New York, p. 437. ACM Press, April 2006
39. Howison, M., Trninic, D., Reinholz, D., Abrahamson, D.: The mathematical imagery trainer. In: Proceedings of the 2011 Annual Conference on Human Factors in Computing Systems, CHI 2011, New York, p. 1989. ACM Press, May 2011
40. Josefi, O.: Non-directive play therapy for young children with autism: a case study. Clin. Child Psychol. Psychiatry **9**(4), 533–551 (2004)
41. Ke, F., Im, T.: Virtual-reality-based social interaction training for children with high-functioning autism. J. Educ. Res. **106**(6), 441–461 (2013)
42. LeGoff, D.B.: Use of LEGO as a therapeutic medium for improving social competence. J. Autism Dev. Disord. **34**(5), 557–571 (2004)
43. MacDonald, M., Lord, C., Ulrich, D.A.: Motor skills and calibrated autism severity in young children with autism spectrum disorder. Adap. Phys. Act. Quart. **31**(2), 95–105 (2014)
44. Macintosh, K., Dissanayake, C.: Social skills and problem behaviours in school aged children with high-functioning autism and asperger's disorder. J. Autism Dev. Disord. **36**(8), 1065–1076 (2006)
45. Malinverni, L., Mora-Guiard, J., Padillo, V., Mairena, M., Hervás, A., Pares, N.: Participatory design strategies to enhance the creative contribution of children with special needs. In: Proceedings of the 2014 Conference on Interaction Design and Children, IDC 2014, New York, pp. 85–94. ACM Press, June 2014
46. Malinverni, L., Mora-Guiard, J., Pares, N.: Towards methods for evaluating and communicating participatory design: a multimodal approach. Int. J. Hum. Comput. Stud. **94**, 53–63 (2016)
47. Malone, T.W.: Heuristics for designing enjoyable user interfaces. In: Proceedings of the 1982 Conference on Human Factors in Computing Systems, CHI 1982, New York, pp. 63–68. ACM Press, March 1982
48. Marwecki, S., Rädle, R., Reiterer, H.: Encouraging collaboration in hybrid therapy games for autistic children. In: CHI 2013 Extended Abstracts on Human Factors in Computing Systems on CHI EA 2013, New York, p. 469. ACM Press, April 2013

49. Mirenda, P.: Toward functional augmentative and alternative communication for students with autism. Lang. Speech Hear. Serv. Schools **34**(3), 203 (2003)
50. Mora-Guiard, J., Crowell, C., Pares, N., Heaton, P.: Lands of fog: helping children with autism in social interaction through a full-body interactive experience. In: ACM SIGCHI Interaction Design and Children 2016 (2016)
51. Morrison, A., Viller, S., Mitchell, P.: Open-ended art environments motivate participation. In: Proceedings of the 8th International Conference on Advances in Computer Entertainment Technology, ACE 2011, pp. 1–8 (2011)
52. Myers, D.: A Q-study of game player aesthetics. Simul. Gaming **21**(4), 375–396 (1990)
53. Neal, L.: Implications of computer games for system design, pp. 93–99, August 1990
54. Parsons, S., Cobb, S.: State-of-the-art of virtual reality technologies for children on the autism spectrum. Eur. J. Spec. Needs Educ. **26**(3), 355–366 (2011)
55. Parsons, S., Leonard, A., Mitchell, P.: Virtual environments for social skills training: comments from two adolescents with autistic spectrum disorder. Comput. Educ. **47**, 186–206 (2006)
56. Rambusch, J., Ziemke, T.: The role of embodiment in situated learning. In: Proceedings of the 27th Annual Conference of the Cognitive Science Society, pp. 1803–1808. Lawrence Erlbaum, Mahwah (2005)
57. Read, J.C., MacFarlane, S.: Using the fun toolkit and other survey methods to gather opinions in child computer interaction. In: Proceeding of the 2006 Conference on Interaction Design and Children, IDC 2006, p. 81 (2006)
58. Revelle, G.: Applying developmental theory and research to the creation of educational games. New Dir. Child Adolesc. Dev. **2013**(139), 31–40 (2013)
59. Rincover, A.: Variables affecting stimulus fading and discriminative responding in psychotic children. J. Abnorm. Psychol. **87**(5), 541–553 (1978)
60. Rowland, C.M., Schweigert, P.D.: Object lessons: how children with autism spectrum disorders use objects to interact with the physical and social environments. Res. Autism Spectr. Disord. **3**(2), 517–527 (2009)
61. Strickland, D.: A virtual reality application with autistic children. Presence Teleoperators Virtual Environ. **5**(3), 319–329 (1996)
62. Strickland, D.C., McAllister, D., Coles, C.D., Osborne, S.: An evolution of virtual reality training designs for children with autism and fetal alcohol spectrum disorders. Topics Lang. Disord. **27**(3), 226–241 (2007)
63. Tager-Flusberg, H., Joseph, R.M.: Identifying neurocognitive phenotypes in autism. Philos. Trans. R. Soc. Lond. Ser. B Biol. Sci. **358**(1430), 303–314 (2003)
64. Trepagnier, C.: Virtual environments for the investigation and rehabilitation of cognitive and perceptual impairments. Neurorehabilitation **12**(1), 63–72 (1999)
65. van Ommeren, T.B., Begeer, S., Scheeren, A.M., Koot, H.M.: Measuring reciprocity in high functioning children and adolescents with autism spectrum disorders. J. Autism Dev. Disord. **42**(6), 1001–1010 (2011)
66. Wieder, S., Greenspan, S.I.: Climbing the symbolic ladder in the DIR model through floor time/interactive play. Autism Int. J. Res. Pract. **7**(4), 425–435 (2003)
67. Zachor, D.A., Ben Itzchak, E.: Treatment approach, autism severity and intervention outcomes in young children. Res. Autism Spectr. Disord. **4**(3), 425–432 (2010)
68. Zarin, R.: Trollskogen: a multitouch table top framework for enhancing communication amongst cognitively disabled children. In: Proceedings of the ACM International Conference on Interactive Tabletops and Surfaces, ITS 2009, p. 1. ACM Press, New York, November 2009

# Stress Detection from Speech
# Using Spectral Slope Measurements

Olympia Simantiraki[1(✉)], Giorgos Giannakakis[1], Anastasia Pampouchidou[2],
and Manolis Tsiknakis[1,3]

[1] Institute of Computer Science, Foundation for Research
and Technology–Hellas (FORTH–ICS), Heraklion, Crete, Greece
{osimantir,tsiknaki}@ics.forth.gr
[2] Le2i Laboratory, University of Burgundy, Le Creusot, France
[3] Department of Informatics Engineering,
Technological Educational Institute of Crete, Heraklion, Crete, Greece

**Abstract.** Automatic detection of emotional stress is an active research domain, which has recently drawn increasing attention, mainly in the fields of computer science, linguistics, and medicine. In this study, stress is automatically detected by employing speech-derived features. Related studies utilize features such as overall intensity, MFCCs, Teager Energy Operator, and pitch. The present study proposes a novel set of features based on the spectral tilt of the glottal source and of the speech signal itself. The proposed features rely on the Probability Density Function of the estimated spectral slopes, and consist of the three most probable slopes from the glottal source, as well as the corresponding three slopes of the speech signal, obtained on a word level. The performance of the proposed method is evaluated on the simulated dataset of the SUSAS corpus, achieving recognition accuracy of 92.06%, when the Random Forests classifier is used.

**Keywords:** Stress detection · Speech analysis · Glottal source
Fundamental frequency · Spectral tilt
Iterative adaptive inverse filtering · Random forests

## 1 Introduction

Automatic detection of stress from speech is of great interest, since speech is considered a significant modality in evaluating stress [1]. Although there is no single agreed definition on speech under stress, it can be referred as *"Stress is observable variability in certain speech features due to a combination of unconscious response to stressors and/or conscious control"* [2]. Automatic stress detection concerns several disciplines such as computer science, linguistics, and medicine. The importance of detecting stress automatically lies in the high prevalence of stress in the modern lifestyle [3], enfolding a wide range of applications from cockpit electronics to polygraph testing, health care, robotics, interactive voice

© ICST Institute for Computer Sciences, Social Informatics and Telecommunications Engineering 2018
N. Oliver et al. (Eds.): MindCare 2016/Fabulous 2016/IIoT 2015, LNICST 207, pp. 41–50, 2018.
https://doi.org/10.1007/978-3-319-74935-8_5

response systems in call-center applications, and in Human Computer Interfaces (HCIs). Such a system could be very valuable in prioritizing emergency calls in hospital/support line call centers where evaluating the severity of each case may be very critical.

The important contribution of human speech in stress assessment has been proved by several studies (e.g., [4]). Speech is a natural human expression in communication. Some features derived from speech (e.g., glottal spectral slope) are more difficult to be manipulated than others (e.g., pitch, intensity). The elicited speech is affected by the speaker's emotions, since emotions affect the muscle tension, which in turn impacts the vortex-flow interaction pattern in the vocal tract [5]. Although in some cases no noticeable effect is observed, there are many cases where speech alteration under stress is significant and easily perceived. The level of change in speech production depends on the intensity and type of emotion expressed (e.g., anger, fear) and/or the environmental conditions the speaker is located into (e.g., Lombard effect [6]). Other studies focus on stress detection using facial cues derived from eyes, mouth, head behavior and camera based heart activity [7]. Additionally, the combination of audio and visual features has proven profitable for emotion recognition [8].

Overall intensity, Teager Energy Operator (TEO), Mel-Frequency Cepstral Coefficients (MFCCs), and functionals of the fundamental frequency ($f_0$), are among the most widely adopted features for detecting speech under stress [9]. The influence of stress in speech is evident, as signals derived from high stressed speech result in greater amplitude of the (glottal) waveform, and more asymmetrical glottal pulse as compared to neutral condition. These changes have an impact on the intensity of the spectrum; it is shifted over the spectrum, and concentrated in the higher frequencies. The literature shows that the relative overall energy of the spectrum increases in a stressed condition; however this is not a sufficient indicator on its own. The distribution and/or spectral tilt of the spectrum's energy has also to be considered, as suggested in [10].

In the present study, metrics based on the spectral tilt are examined, proving the significant role of spectral tilt in discriminating stressed from neutral speech with high accuracy. Feature extraction is performed using the simulated dataset of the SUSAS corpus [11]. In order to validate the reliability of the proposed features, the statistical test Mann–Whitney is used, which revealed a statistically significant difference between the stressed and neutral indicators and the Random Forests are used for the classification.

## 2   Related Work

Several studies have focused on the detection of emotional stress from speech, highlighting the distinctive differences in phonation between stressed and neutral speech [12]. Feature analysis methods for classification of speech under stress have also been proposed [9]. Most studies use simulated stressed speech data for evaluation [13] with specific utterances usually being isolated for the analysis [12,14]. A notable limitation of the latter is that the results degrade as the test conditions drift from the environmental or experimental conditions of the training data [12].

A review of available literature showed that the most widely studied features for discriminating neutral and stressed speech are: overall intensity, TEO, MFCCs and functionals of the fundamental frequency (mainly standard deviation, mean and variance) [9]. *Shah et al.* [15] employed Discrete Wavelet Transform (DWT) for feature extraction, and Artificial Neural Networks (ANN) for classification, achieving 85% recognition accuracy. In *Godin et al.* [9], 6 glottal features were extracted, while Gaussian Mixture Model (GMM) was used as the classifier, achieving detection accuracy of 69%. *Sondhi et al.* [16] suggested to use the mean pitch and the formants (F1, F2) of the human voice as reliable and non-invasive indicators of emotional stress, since they were the acoustic measures providing the most significant change under stress. Eleven subjects participated in this study, providing answers from a specific set of responses: "yes", "no", "haan" ("haan" means "yes" in Hindi language). In [12], TEO based features were extracted and Hidden Markov Model (HMM) was used for the stressed speech classifier. The classification error rate for the stress/neutral speech was 4.7/4.6% for the closed-speaker-set system, and 13.6/4.0% for the open-speaker-set system. *Fernandez* and *Picard* [17] explored the use of a feature set based on subband decompositions and the TEO. The corpus used consisted of 598 short speech utterances collected from four subjects driving in a simulator. The best performance obtained, with the speaker-dependent mixture model, achieved an accuracy of 96.4% on the training set, and of 61.2% on a separate testing set. Also, the authors concluded that the performance of the speaker-independent model degrades with respect to the models trained on individual speakers.

A second group of studies [13], have underlined the spectrum significance for discriminating stressed and neutral speech characteristics. *Shukla et al.* [13] extracted the Relative Formant Peak Displacement (RFD) and MFCCs, as features for neutral and stressed speech separation. The simulated speech data (neutral, angry, sad and Lombard) used for evaluation was in Hindi and Indian language. A HMM was used, and the combination of RFD and MFCC achieved 59.53% accuracy. In [18], articulatory, excitation (pitch, duration, intensity) and cepstral based features were estimated using the SUSAS database and an HMM classifier achieving an accuracy of 80.6%.

A different approach was proposed by *Yao et al.* [14], where physical characteristics of the vocal folds were investigated. A novel metric, namely the Muscle Tension Ratio (MTR) was introduced to identify speech under stress. Vowel instances /a/ were isolated for the analysis and ROC curves were used for evaluating and comparing the classification of MTR with the Spectral Flatness Measure (SFM), a conversational method of stress measurement. Experimental results showed that MTR outperforms the conversational method of stress measurement.

Drawn from the reported review of literature, SUSAS is among the most widely employed databases used in defining metrics for the automatic discrimination of stressed and neutral speech. Due to the overt variances in the speech and glottal spectrum of stressed and unstressed speech, the features selected for the investigation in this work are based on spectrum variance.

## 3   Dataset

As already mentioned, the speech corpus used in this study is the widely used, simulated dataset of SUSAS [11]. It consists of 9 male speakers, uttering isolated-words (e.g., "break", "enter", "change") in a quiet environment. The recordings used are 70 words per speaker, pronounced in four styles: neutral, angry, loud, and Lombard effect. In this study only these three stress types are used as they are the most common employed stress conditions [5]. Speech samples are separated into two general clusters: (a) unstressed speech cluster consisting of the neutral utterances (b) stressed speech cluster consisting of the angry, loud, and Lombard utterances. The total number of samples is 630 words of unstressed speech and 1890 words of stressed speech. The speech tokens were sampled in a 16-bit A/D converter with 8 kHz sampling rate.

## 4   Feature Extraction

In the speech production model, the acoustic speech signal is the result of the glottal source signal[1] modulated by a transfer (filter) function, the vocal tract. Equation (1), shows mathematically this convolution process

$$s[n] = g[n] \star v[n] \tag{1}$$

where $s[n]$ is the speech signal derived from the convolution of the impulse response of the vocal tract $v[n]$ with the glottal source excitation signal $g[n]$. When a speaker is under stress, both the vocal folds and the movement of the articulators (vocal tract) are affected. Therefore, for a reliable detection of stressed speech, features based on the glottal source signal and speech characteristics should be taken into consideration. In human speech, stressed syllables are produced with greater vocal effort. If a speaker makes greater vocal effort, the amplitudes of the higher frequencies increase more than that of the lower frequencies [19]. For this reason, the use of the spectral tilt is introduced as a measure of the relative distribution of spectral energy from lower to higher frequencies [20]. The proposed features are computed both for the output-speech signal and for the glottal source signal. Furthermore, the standard deviation of the fundamental frequency is extracted, since it has been proven to be a good feature for the separation of stressed and neutral speech [21]. In this study, the analysis of the extracted features is performed only on the voiced speech areas which are discriminated using the $f_0$ estimation from the SWIPE algorithm [22].

---

[1] Glottal source signal is the signal generated at the glottis which could be either periodic pulses or noise.

## 4.1    Fundamental Frequency

The fundamental frequency ($f_0$) has been widely used in several studies (e.g., [23]) and has proven to be a good indicator for separating stressed from neutral speech. As already mentioned, in this study, the fundamental frequency is estimated only for the voiced areas using the SWIPE algorithm [22] and its standard deviation was selected as the feature to be used in the subsequent analysis. The pitch is searched within a specific range ([70 450] in Herz) and is estimated every 5 ms. The $f_0$ has been normalized in the range [0, 1].

## 4.2    Spectral Slopes

In estimating the spectral slopes, the voiced areas are isolated using the $f_0$ estimation from the SWIPE algorithm. No estimation is made in the unvoiced areas, and thus these frames are excluded from the analysis. Then, the magnitude spectrum is computed using the Fast Fourier Transform (FFT) with 30 ms window length and 5 ms overlap. The spectral envelope [24] is subsequently estimated with optimal spectral order computed by $\lfloor \frac{f_s}{2f_0} \rfloor$ (where $f_s$ is the sampling frequency and $f_0$ is the fundamental frequency) normalized in dB. Finally, in order to compute the spectral tilt, a linear regression line is fitted to the spectral envelope of the frame using the least square error method and the slope of the regression line is obtained as a measure for the spectral tilt. The same procedure is repeated for all voiced segments of each word. The probability density function (PDF) is computed for each word for the bag-of-slopes extracted (one slope per voiced frame). Then, the three most probable slopes of PDF histogram are used as features for the classification. The bin width in the histogram is 0.017 (this value corresponds to $\pi/180$ rad).

**Glottal Source Signal.** During stressed phonation, a combination of changes in sub-glottal air pressure can lead to irregular shape of the glottal pulses [25]. In Fig. 1, the glottal pulses for the stressed speech (angry) and neutral speech are depicted. In order to estimate the glottal source signal, we employed the Iterative Adaptive Inverse Filtering (IAIF) method [26] using linear prediction for the estimation of the vocal tract response. The IAIF removes the vocal tract effects in an iterative manner in order to obtain an accurate estimation of the glottal source signal. The observed differences are also reflected on the glottal spectrum, resulting in increased energy at higher frequency areas. The mean glottal spectrums and the corresponding spectral tilts, computed on the same voiced part for each condition, i.e. stressed and neutral, are illustrated in Fig. 2(a), in which differences can be clearly observed. Based on the observation regarding the characteristics of the spectrum, feature extraction based on the spectral tilt of the glottal source spectrum is proposed herein. In Fig. 2(b), the PDF of the spectral tilt for the voiced tokens of the spoken word /NAV/, for both stressed and unstressed speech styles are shown. The three highest peaks of the PDF curves for each word are selected for the classification. Additionally, in Fig. 2(b),

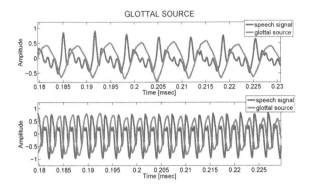

**Fig. 1.** *Upper panel*: a neutral speech segment (*blue line*) and its corresponding glottal source (*red line*). *Lower panel*: a stressed (angry) speech signal (*blue line*) and its corresponding glottal source (*red line*). Token /a/ is uttered by a male speaker in both panels, isolated from the word /NAV/. (Color figure online)

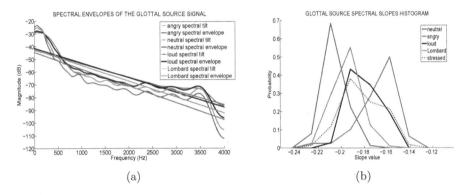

**Fig. 2.** (a) *Solid lines*: mean values of the glottal source spectral envelopes. *Dashed lines*: corresponding spectral tilts. (b) Probability Density Functions of the glottal spectral slopes. All information is extracted from the voiced tokens isolated from the word /NAV/ uttered by a male speaker, for neutral speech (*blue solid line*), 3 different stressed speech styles (*red, black, magenta solid lines*), and the combined stressed speech styles (*blue dashed line*). (Color figure online)

we observe that the PDF curve of the stressed speech is to the right of the neutral curve, which means that the glottal spectrum tilt of the stressed speech is greater than that of the neutral. Most commonly, if the glottal waveshape is less smooth, it will have a stronger harmonic structure and a spectral slope closer to zero [9], as opposed to neutral speech, for which the spectral slope for voiced frames is typically negative.

**Speech Signal.** A stressed speaker utilizes a more pronounced and loud voice, changing the shape of the vocal tract formants. More precisely, in a condition of stress the location of the formants and their bandwidth are different than in neutral speech [21,25]. Also the filter function is excited by the source spectrum, resulting in a tilt in the overall spectrum. The stress affects higher frequency regions more than that of the lower frequency regions. Therefore, under stress conditions, the spectral tilt increases with respect to neutral condition (Fig. 3(a)). As the spectrum of the speech signal could enhance the glottal spectrum information, the speech spectral slope is also prominent for characterization and classification of stressed speech. The three highest peaks in the PDF curve (Fig. 3(b)) for each word are used as additional features for the classification.

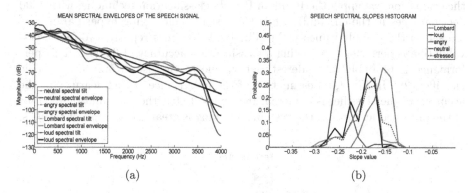

(a)    (b)

**Fig. 3.** (a) *Solid lines*: mean values of the speech signal spectral envelopes. *Dashed lines*: corresponding spectral tilts. (b) Probability Density Functions of the speech signal spectral slopes. All information is extracted from the voiced tokens isolated from the word /NAV/ uttered by a male subject, for neutral speech (*blue solid line*), 3 different stressed speech styles (*red, black, magenta solid lines*), and the combined stressed speech styles (*blue dashed line*). (Color figure online)

# 5 Statistical and Classification Analysis

The statistically significant difference between the stressed and neutral PDF curves, from which the spectrum based features have been extracted, is quantified with the statistical test Mann–Whitney. Figures 2(b) and 3(b), illustrate this significant difference of the distributions resulting from the spectral tilt of stressed and neutral speech. Two separate Mann–Whitney statistical tests are performed. In the first test, the glottal and speech spectral slopes of the neutral style and the corresponding spectral slopes of all stressed styles are compared using the statistical test for each speaker individually. The individual difference of the distributions is statistically significant ($p < 0.01$). In the second test, the same statistical test is performed between the neutral and stressed spectral slopes (glottal and speech slopes separately) for all nine speakers yielding statistically significant differentiation between the distributions ($p < 0.01$). Based on the reported findings, the spectral slopes can be characterized as significant informative indicators for distinguishing neutral from stressed speech.

The Random Forests (RF) algorithm [27] is applied in order to evaluate the performance of the proposed features (three glottal spectral slopes, three speech spectral slopes, and the standard deviation of the $f_0$), for the discrimination between stressed and unstressed speech. The RF is an aggregation of decision trees algorithm. This method is considered as a general technique of decision trees, and is an ensemble learning method for classification. The main advantage of the Random Forests algorithm, is that it corrects the decision trees' tendency of over-fitting to their training set. More specifically, a text-independent classification is performed using all of the 2520 recordings from the SUSAS dataset. For the evaluation, we apply the Random Forests classification technique, with 1000 decision trees in the ensemble, while the rest of their tuning hyper-parameters are set to the default values in MATLAB. A 10 times repeated 10-fold cross-validation is performed, achieving a classification accuracy of 92.06%. This performance is probably an underestimation due to the use of only one specific classifier [28]. In Fig. 4, an estimation of the importance of each feature for the accuracy of the classifier is depicted. It is evident that the contribution of three of the proposed features in the system's learning is greater than that of the $f_0$'s.

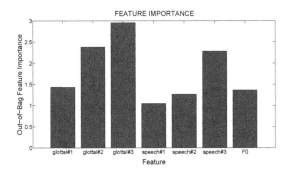

**Fig. 4.** Proposed features are denoted with the labels *glottal#1, glottal#2, glottal#3, speech#1, speech#2, speech#3 (glottal#n are the 3 most probable glottal spectral slopes provided by the PDF histogram and speech#n the corresponding speech spectral slopes)* and with *F0* the $f_0$ std.

## 6   Conclusion

This study focuses on separating the neutral from stressed speech, using features estimated on the frequency domain. More specifically, the features used are the three most probable slopes of the speech spectrum provided by the PDF histogram, the corresponding three slopes of the glottal spectrum, and the standard deviation of the $f_0$. These features are extracted for the voiced segments of each word in the dataset and not for specific tokens. The main advantage of the proposed features is that they cannot be easily manipulated for concealing stress, in contrast to the most commonly used features in similar studies, e.g., overall intensity and pitch, which can be voluntarily controlled. Therefore they form the basis for a more objective estimation method. Furthermore, it is not sufficient to deal only with the overall intensity, since a shift of the intensity over the spectrum is observed when more effort is made for the speech production. This shift is apparent on the spectral tilt. In this study, the classification performed using the metrics based on spectral tilt and $f_0$ was text-independent achieving an accuracy score of 92.06%. As a result, our main conclusion is that these metrics are capable of distinguishing the two speaking styles with great success.

Future work will focus on extended data analysis by testing different classifiers, on applying the proposed features on datasets with stressed and neutral recordings under real conditions and on evaluating the detection accuracy by combining these speech features with visual features, in an analysis approach similar to the one in [29].

**Acknowledgments.** The authors acknowledge support from the iManageCancer EU project under contract H2020-PHC-26-2014 No.643529.

# References

1. Sharma, N., Gedeon, T.: Objective measures, sensors and computational techniques for stress recognition and classification: A survey. Comput. Methods Programs Biomed. **108**(3), 1287–1301 (2012)
2. Murray, I.R., Baber, C., South, A.: Towards a definition and working model of stress and its effects on speech. Speech Commun. **20**(1), 3–12 (1996)
3. Selye, H.: The Stress of Life. McGraw-Hill, New York (1956)
4. Lefter, I., Rothkrantz, L.J., Van Leeuwen, D.A., Wiggers, P.: Automatic stress detection in emergency (telephone) calls. Int. J. Intell. Defence Support Syst. **4**(2), 148–168 (2011)
5. Zhou, G.J., Hansen, J.H.L., Kaiser, J.F.: Nonlinear feature based classification of speech under stress. IEEE Trans. Speech Audio Process. **9**(3), 201–216 (2001)
6. Garnier, M., Henrich, N.: Speaking in noise: How does the Lombard effect improve acoustic contrasts between speech and ambient noise? Comput. Speech Lang. **28**(2), 580–597 (2014)
7. Giannakakis, G., Pediaditis, M., Manousos, D., Kazantzaki, E., Chiarugi, F., Simos, P.G., Marias, K., Tsiknakis, M.: Stress and anxiety detection using facial cues from videos. Biomed. Signal Process. Control **31**, 89–101 (2017)
8. Zeng, Z., Pantic, M., Roisman, G.I., Huang, T.S.: A survey of affect recognition methods: Audio, visual, and spontaneous expressions. IEEE Trans. Pattern Anal. Mach. Intell. **31**, 39–58 (2009)
9. Godin, K.W., Hasan, T., Hansen, J.H.: Glottal waveform analysis of physical task stress speech. In: INTERSPEECH, pp. 1648–1651 (2012)
10. Sluijter, A.M., Van Heuven, V.J.: Spectral balance as an acoustic correlate of linguistic stress. J. Acoust. Soc. Am. **100**(4), 2471–2485 (1996)
11. Hansen, J.H., Bou-Ghazale, S.E., Sarikaya, R., Pellom, B.: Getting started with SUSAS: a speech under simulated and actual stress database. In: Eurospeech, vol. 97(4), pp. 1743–46 (1997)

12. Hansen, J.H., Kim, W., Rahurkar, M., Ruzanski, E., Meyerhoff, J.: Robust emotional stressed speech detection using weighted frequency subbands. EURASIP J. Adv. Signal Process. **2011**(1), 1–10 (2011)
13. Shukla, S., Dandapat, S., Prasanna, S.R.M.: Spectral slope based analysis and classification of stressed speech. Int. J. Speech Technol. **14**(3), 245–258 (2011)
14. Yao, X., Jitsuhiro, T., Miyajima, C., Kitaoka, N., Takeda, K.: Physical characteristics of vocal folds during speech under stress. In: IEEE International Conference on Acoustics, Speech and Signal Processing (ICASSP), pp. 4609–4612 (2012)
15. Shah, F., Sukumar, R., Anto, B.: Automatic Stress Detection from Speech by Using Discrete Wavelet Transforms (2009)
16. Sondhi, S., Khan, M., Vijay, R., Salhan, A.K.: Vocal indicators of emotional stress. Int. J. Comput. Appl. **122**(15), 38–43 (2015)
17. Fernandez, R., Rosalind, W.P.: Modeling drivers speech under stress. Speech Commun. **40**(1), 145–159 (2003)
18. Womak, B.D., Hansen, J.H.: Improved speech recognition via speaker stress directed classification. In: IEEE International Conference on Acoustics, Speech, and Signal Processing, ICASSP, vol. 1, pp. 53–56 (1996)
19. Eriksson, A., Traunmüller, H.: Perception of vocal effort and distance from the speaker on the basis of vowel utterances. Percept. Psychophysics **64**(1), 131–139 (2002)
20. Tartter, V.C., Gomes, H., Litwin, E.: Some acoustic effects of listening to noise on speech production. J. Acoust. Soc. Am. **94**(4), 2437–2440 (1993)
21. Sigmund, M.: Introducing the database ExamStress for speech under stress. In: Proceedings of the 7th Nordic Signal Processing Symposium-NORSIG, pp. 290–293. IEEE (2006)
22. Camacho, A.: SWIPE: A sawtooth waveform inspired pitch estimator for speech and music. Doctoral dissertation, University of Florida (2007)
23. Protopapas, A., Lieberman, P.: Fundamental frequency of phonation and perceived emotional stress. J. Acoust. Soc. Am. **101**(4), 2267–2277 (1997)
24. Röbel, A., Rodet, X.: Efficient spectral envelope estimation and its application to pitch shifting and envelope preservation. In: International Conference on Digital Audio Effects, pp. 30–35 (2005)
25. Hansen, J.H.L., Patil, S.: Speech under stress: analysis, modeling and recognition. In: Müller, C. (ed.) Speaker Classification I. LNCS (LNAI), vol. 4343, pp. 108–137. Springer, Heidelberg (2007). https://doi.org/10.1007/978-3-540-74200-5_6
26. Alku, P.: Glottal wave analysis with pitch synchronous iterative adaptive inverse filtering. Speech Commun. **11**(2–3), 109–118 (1992)
27. Hastie, T., Tibshirani, R., Friedman, J.: The Elements of Statistical Learning, 2nd edn. Springer, New York (2008)
28. Tsamardinos, I., Rakhshani, A., Lagani, V.: Performance-estimation properties of cross-validation-based protocols with simultaneous hyper-parameter optimization. In: Likas, A., Blekas, K., Kalles, D. (eds.) SETN 2014. LNCS (LNAI), vol. 8445, pp. 1–14. Springer, Cham (2014). https://doi.org/10.1007/978-3-319-07064-3_1
29. Pampouchidou, A., Simantiraki, O., Fazlollahi, A., Pediaditis, M., Manousos, D., Roniotis, A., Giannakakis, G., Meriaudeau, F., Simos, P., Marias, K., Yang, F., Tsiknakis, M.: Depression assessment by fusing high and low level features from audio, video, and text. In: The 6th Audio/Visual Emotion Challenge and Workshop. ACM-Multimedia (2016)

# Technological Devices as an Opportunity for People with Parkinson

Petra Maresova[(✉)]

University of Hradec Kralove, Rokitanskeho 62,
50003 Hradec Kralove, Czech Republic
Petra.maresova@uhk.cz

**Abstract.** The incidence of dementia in developed countries has been incessantly growing. Apart from new medication and medical equipment, a lot of effort is placed on developing modern information technologies. This contribution aims to analyse the areas of current research aimed at technologies supporting those suffering from Parkinson's disease, which is worldwide the second most common type of dementia. Then, it will be specified in what areas modern technologies may help improve care for patients with Parkinson's. The method to conduct this study was literature review of accessible sources in PubMed, Scopus, Web of Science and ScienceDirect databases. The results showed that technologies are beneficial for patients with Parkinson's disease in these areas: better personal health and quality of life; ability to better manage own health; receiving faster and more frequent feedback about one's health; and saving time of caregivers.

**Keywords:** Technology · Mobile application · Parkinson disease
Medical device

## 1 Introduction

Parkinson's disease is one of the most common neurological disorders affecting 60-plus-year-old people. However, rare forms of this disease may develop even before 40 years of age [1]. The risk of developing Parkinson's disease increases with age. As more people reach senior age, the incidence of Parkinson's disease is higher, too [2].

Although pharmacological treatment significantly influences symptoms of the disease, they do not restore lost motor skills. Therefore, treatment includes adjusting daily routines and treatment of gait-related problems. Modern technologies may further improve the state of PD patients. Current assistive technology products involve devices that address specific needs, such as "wayfinding", social interaction, memory support and health management, but to be truly beneficial for dementia sufferers they need to work together in an intelligent way [3]. Technology development is also supported by the fact that 85% would want to stay living in their home if diagnosed with dementia, which would be impossible without either personal assistance or intelligent systems.

This contribution aims to analyse the areas of current research focusing on technologies supporting PD patients and specifies what areas of development may benefit PD patients.

© ICST Institute for Computer Sciences, Social Informatics and Telecommunications Engineering 2018
N. Oliver et al. (Eds.): MindCare 2016/Fabulous 2016/IIoT 2015, LNICST 207, pp. 51–55, 2018.
https://doi.org/10.1007/978-3-319-74935-8_6

## 2  Methods

For the purpose of this study a method of literature review of available sources describing current modern information technologies and their role in the stages of Parkinson's disease was used. The authors worked with databases like PubMed, ScienceDirect, Web of Science and Scopus, where they reviewed original studies linked to their topic on the basis of the keywords "Parkinson's disease AND technology", "Parkinson's disease AND wearables", "Parkinson's disease AND Mobile technology" in the period from 2010 to 2016. First, all duplicities were eliminated. Many results were focused too widely and they were connected with the use of modern technologies in healthcare. In addition, they were connected with different types of dementia or, on the contrary, the articles concentrated exclusively on Parkinson's disease and the issue of technologies was solved only marginally. Therefore, the authors examined only those research studies which were closely connected with the explored topic. The total number of used sources corresponding with these criteria was 21.

## 3  Results and Discussion

Table 1 explores the randomized clinical studies which examine the use and effectiveness of technological devices in the care or treatment of Parkinson's disease. Although the findings from Table 1 are short-term with a small size of subjects, they show that technologies might be beneficial for patients with Parkinson's disease:

- better personal health and quality of life;
- ability to better manage own health;
- receiving faster and more frequent feedback about one's health;
- and saving time of caregivers [3].

The use of these applications should respect the patient's technological knowledge and skills. It remains to be solved how to ensure safety of mobile medical applications, allay fears about the abuse of collected data, and improve interoperability of accessible solutions. There are also problems like:

- protecting and treating sensitive information;
- burden of application;
- impact on clinical care;
- and negative impact on health, reminded cloud cause exacerbation.

**Table 1.** The use of technological devices in the care or treatment of Parkinson's disease

| Study | Subjects, method | Technology | Benefits/limitations |
|---|---|---|---|
| Feasibility and effects of home-based smartphone-delivered automated feedback training for gait in people with Parkinson's disease: a pilot randomized controlled trial [4] | N = 40, training for 30 min, three times per week for six weeks | Inertial measurement units combined with a smartphone application (CuPiD-system) to provide real-time feedback on gait performance | Study describes, that this technology is an effective approach to promote gait training. This benefit may be ascribed to the real-time feedback, stimulating corrective actions and promoting self-efficacy to achieve optimal performance. Further optimization of the system and determining of cost-effectiveness is needed |
| How well do Parkinson's disease patients turn in bed? Quantitative analysis of nocturnal hypokinesia using multisite wearable inertial sensors [5] | N = 19, one night at their homes | Multisite inertial sensors to compare nocturnal movements of PD patients | Study showed that PD patients significantly had fewer rolling over, turned with smaller degree, less velocity, and acceleration, but had more episodes of getting out of bed. For effective treatment strategy should be done a comprehensive review of both day- and nighttime symptoms |
| Analyzing activity behavior and movement in a naturalistic environment using smart home techniques [6] | N = 84, machine learning techniques | Smart home and wearable sensors to collect data about the impact of different medical conditions on daily behavior | Machine learning techniques describes differences between healthy older adults and adults with Parkinson disease. It was confirmed that these differences can be automatically recognized |
| E-health support in people with Parkinson's disease with smart glasses: a survey of user requirements and expectations in the Netherlands [7] | N = 62, 11 months Survey about the requirements, constraints, and attitudes of people with PD to this new technology | Smart glasses | Study confirmed that smart glasses are new therapeutic and monitoring possibility which is well adopted, especially by younger people with PD |
| Wearability assessment of a wearable system for Parkinson's disease remote monitoring based on a body area network of sensors [8] | N = 32, the compliance of a telehealth system for the remote monitoring of Parkinson's disease (PD) patients | Telehealth system for the remote monitoring of Parkinson's disease (PD) patients. This system, called PERFORM, is based on a Body Area Network | The test results showed that the acceptance of this system is satisfactory with all the levels of effect on each component scoring in the lowest ranges |

(*continued*)

**Table 1.** (*continued*)

| Study | Subjects, method | Technology | Benefits/limitations |
|---|---|---|---|
| | | (BAN) of sensors which has already been validated both from the technical and clinical point for view | |
| A wearable proprioceptive stabilizer (Equistasi®) for rehabilitation of postural instability in Parkinson's disease: a phase II randomized double-blind, double-dummy, controlled study [9] | N = 40 (two groups 20 and 20), two months | Wearable proprioceptive stabilizer (Equistasi) that emits focal mechanical vibrations in patients with PD | The potential to be more effectiveness to be superior than rehabilitation alone in improving patients' balance. Small sample |
| Mobile apps for the treatment of depression [10] | Veterans aged 18 and older, Time Frame: Week 1, Week 4, Week 8 | Mood Coach app - Behavioral activation plus mobile app - offer the opportunity for real-time tracking of behavior and have the ability to provide prompt feedback and reminders | Greater adherence to the BA treatment compared to the standard BA condition Greater satisfaction with the app compared to the standard BA protocol that utilizes paper and pencil materials |

**Acknowledgement.** This paper is published thanks to the support of the internal projects Economic and Managerial Aspects of Processes in Biomedicine.

# References

1. Grimes, D.A.: Parkinson's Disease: A Guide to Treatments, Therapies and Controlling Symptoms. Constable & Robinson Ltd., London (2004)
2. Dorsey, E.R., Constantinescu, R., Thompson, J.P., et al.: Projected number of people with Parkinson disease in the most populous nations, 2005 through 2030. Neurology **68**(5), 384–386 (2007)
3. Hall, W.: Technology Could Help People with Dementia Remain in Their Homes. The Guardian (2014)
4. Ginis, P., Nieuwboer, A., Dorfman, M., Ferrari, A., et al.: Feasibility and effects of home-based smartphone-delivered automated feedback training for gait in people with Parkinson's disease: a pilot randomized controlled trial. Parkinsonism Relat. Disord. **15**, 30027-4 (2015). https://doi.org/10.1016/j.parkreldis.2015.11.004
5. Sringean, J., Taechalertpaisarn, P., Thanawattano, C., Bhidayasiri, R.: How well do Parkinson's disease patients turn in bed? Quantitative analysis of nocturnal hypokinesia using multisite wearable inertial sensors. Parkinsonism Relat. Disord. **23**, 10–16 (2016). https://doi.org/10.1016/j.parkreldis.2015.11.003

6. Cook, D.J., Schmitter-Edgecombe, M., Dawadi, P.: Analyzing activity behavior and movement in a naturalistic environment using smart home techniques. IEEE J. Biomed. Health Inform. **19**(6), 1882–1892 (2015). https://doi.org/10.1109/JBHI.2015.2461659
7. Zhao, Y., Heida, T., van Wegen, E.E., Bloem, B.R., van Wezel, R.J.: E-health support in people with Parkinson's disease with smart glasses: a survey of user requirements and expectations in the Netherlands. J. Parkinsons Dis. **5**(2), 369–378 (2015). https://doi.org/10. 3233/jpd150568
8. Cancela, J., Pastorino, M., Tzallas, A.T., et al.: Wearability assessment of a wearable system for Parkinson's disease remote monitoring based on a body area network of sensors. Sensors (Basel) **14**(9), 17235–17255 (2014). https://doi.org/10.3390/s140917235
9. Volpe, D., Giantin, M.G., Fasano, A.: A wearable proprioceptive stabilizer (Equistasi®) for rehabilitation of postural instability in Parkinson's disease: a phase II randomized double-blind, double-dummy, controlled study. PLoS One. **9**(11), e112065 (2014). https:// doi.org/10.1371/journal.pone.0112065
10. Lejuez, C.W., Hopko, D.R., Acierno, R., Daughters, S.B., Pagoto, S.L.: Ten year revision of the brief behavioral activation treatment for depression: revised treatment manual. Behav. Modif. **35**(2), 111–161 (2011). https://doi.org/10.1177/0145445510390929

# just Physio kidding - NUI and Gamification based Therapeutic Intervention for Children with Special Needs

Rui Neves Madeira[1(⊠)] ⓘ, André Antunes[1],
and Octavian Postolache[2]

[1] Escola Superior de Tecnologia de Setúbal, IPS, Setúbal, Portugal
rui.madeira@estsetubal.ips.pt,
andre.punk.antunes@gmail.com
[2] Instituto de Telecomunicações and ISCTE-IUL, Lisbon, Portugal
opostolache@lx.it.pt

**Abstract.** This paper presents the "just Physio kidding" approach, which intends to improve the engaging qualities of therapy programmes towards children with special needs, mainly with cerebral palsy, spinal muscular atrophy, or developmental delay. Therefore, "just Physio kidding" intends to address both physiotherapy and cognitive stimulation therapy. The system is functioning as a complement to the work of therapists, with and without their live supervision. It is part of a project with the aim of developing software based on the concept of personalized serious games for rehabilitation. The paper presents the concept and the prototype behind "just Physio kidding".

**Keywords:** Natural User Interface · NUI · Physiotherapy · Serious games
Children with special needs · Cognitive stimulation · Cerebral palsy
Gamification

## 1 Introduction and Background

Recent years have seen a healthcare community demonstrating much interest in therapy approaches based on serious games (theragames) to improve the engaging qualities of its programmes [1]. Gamification [2] can provide rehabilitation environments that can increase the motivation of patients to achieve successful completion of rehabilitation programs that can be dreary or very demanding [3]. Several projects based on theragames have appeared, which shows a wide general interest in sustaining and improving this technology towards a more versatile and wide-range therapy. The utility of this technology is demonstrated by projects in diverse areas, which for instance can work as means of increasing compliance or help patients follow through with otherwise often-repetitive therapy tasks [4, 5]. Among the theragames, exergames are a form of physical activity that requires the user to move at least a part of the body in order to interact and best experience the game. These exergames are considered active games with the goal of creating stimulating methods to maintain an active lifestyle tailored to the specific physiological and psychological conditions of patients, thus being designed

© ICST Institute for Computer Sciences, Social Informatics and Telecommunications Engineering 2018
N. Oliver et al. (Eds.): MindCare 2016/Fabulous 2016/IIoT 2015, LNICST 207, pp. 56–61, 2018.
https://doi.org/10.1007/978-3-319-74935-8_7

explicitly to help them improve their physical health [6]. Exergames have been successfully applied to the rehabilitation of people with motor impairments [6].

Moreover, in the last decade, the use of Virtual Reality (VR) technologies has expanded rapidly for creating innovative tools for rehabilitation. VR-based rehabilitation uses sensing devices to capture and quantitatively assess the movements of patients that are under treatment to track their progress more accurately [7]. A 3D camera is one of those sensing devices, which combined with serious games turns out to be a perspective tool in advanced rehabilitation sessions. The development of more cost-effective devices, such as Microsoft Kinect, means that the development of Natural User Interfaces (NUI) is gaining a wider space and great importance across all fields. NUI can be seen as the ability to interact with a machine using nothing but the human body, avoiding the use of visible control elements to the greatest possible extent to ensure a more natural control. Thus, the use of Microsoft Kinect to control the games, provide feedback to patients, and even as a measuring tool, is a valuable asset to the rehabilitation process among different projects [7, 8]. The integration of VR and NUI technologies with exergames can provide more motivation and engagement to patients while they are in rehabilitation activities [7].

We conducted a previous study [9] to assess the importance of using gamification and NUI-based devices, such as Kinect, in physiotherapy. A survey was directed exclusively to physiotherapists that work mainly with victims of stroke, older adults, and children with special needs that present reduced mobility. The large majority of participants stated patients were highly motivated to use these solutions. Motivation was, indeed, the argument most frequently mentioned, but others arguments were that they could be a valuable complement to physiotherapy and they could be strongly directed to the younger patients. In order to better complement classic physiotherapy, participants also expected monitoring and feedback capabilities from these solutions.

Therefore, we are creating an interactive and smart rehabilitation exergaming system by exploiting the concepts of gamification and NUI. This paper presents "just Physio kidding" (jPk), which applies the findings from our previous work, aiming to encourage physical exercise in order to combat physical deterioration while working on the cognitive stimulation component. It should be a complement to the therapists that work with children with special needs, especially with cerebral palsy (CP).

## 2   The "just Physio kidding" Prototype

### 2.1   Principles

The main idea behind "just Physio kidding" is the implementation of a richly interactive and smart rehabilitation exergaming system towards each one of its users (patients and therapists). Moreover, we are exploiting the use of NUI devices and, in a first phase, we started by using Microsoft Kinect to infer mechanical motion of patients since it is a relatively low-cost consumer game interface device and easy to set up. The project was then designed having in mind the therapy work in a clinic that deals with children with special needs, such as the cases of children with spinal muscular atrophy or developmental delay, besides the ones with CP.

For instance, CP is a group of disorders that affects the development of movement and posture, causing activity limitations [10]. Children with CP have muscle weakness, reduced range of motion, and poor control over their movements, which pose additional difficulties and challenges with the finely controlled movement required by Kinect [6]. This way, it is required to provide a high motivation to these children to comply with crucial treatments and therapies. The gamification of these therapies' exercises and their deployment in ubiquitous and NUI based devices may provide a more engaging and compelling rehabilitation [11], even at patients' homes with the supervision of the parents. However, the implementation of jPk needs to take into account both the specific context being gamified and the qualities of the end-users [11], the children with special needs, in order to obtain the desired outcomes.

Therefore, jPk relies on the Gamification and NUI concepts in order to encourage physical exercise to combat both physical and cognitive deterioration, and it should function as a complement to the work of therapists, with and without their real-time supervision. The therapist plays an important role in this system since s/he is the user responsible for (1) configuring the jPk's components according to each patient's needs; (2) supervising patients' performance and progress. Besides the patients (children) and the therapists, jPk also presents the role of administrator as a third user. This user is the responsible for the whole system, issuing general reports and supervising the jPk installations in clinics and others spaces. Figure 1 shows the different components and their connections. It should be noted that the patient has access to the NUI-based gaming component (JPK), and the therapist has access to the JPKT component that presents two interfaces: a NUI-based interface that allows the therapist to configure and supervise her/his patients' sessions in loco, in the therapy clinic's scenario, and a Web interface which is focused on providing remote access to a wider range of configurations and more detailed dashboards about patients' results and progress.

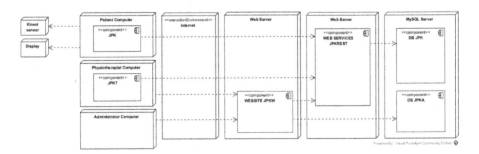

**Fig. 1.** The physical architecture of "just Physio kidding".

Based on previous findings [9], the jPk team's therapists have selected an initial set of essential basic movements (Table 1) of the upper-body, more specifically of the upper-limb, for balance training and motor coordination. The basis of the core game mechanics of jPk is based on these movements since they are crucial for the rehabilitation process of the patients targeted by jPk.

**Table 1.** The set of essential basic movements.

| Movement | Description |
| --- | --- |
| Weight transfer | Transferring the weight of the body from one hip to another |
| Side reach | Inclination of the trunk - for both sides |
| Anterior reach | Take torso forward |
| Rotation of the trunk | For both sides |
| Later reach | Bring torso back |

In a first therapy scenario of jPk, we have one display and a Kinect device for each user, all of them connected to the same computer (middle server). Each display will show its application running. In a second scenario, there is only one Kinect and one display connected to the home computer, for instance. In both scenarios, data will be sent to the jPk's server in order to be processed and integrated into a global view. This allows having appropriate supervision, even when we have a patient that is in her/his home or doing rehabilitation exercises more independently in the clinic.

## 2.2 Gaming and User Interfaces

Since the jPk system is based on PhysioMate [9], it is composed of two different sets of NUI-based serious games: routines and challenges. Regarding the routines set, the patient plays games that are routines of movements created by the physiotherapist. The main aspects of this game are the following: directed only for physiotherapy, there can be scheduled routines that integrate a global plan of rehabilitation exercises created by the therapist, who can, for instance, create and add routines to the system, supervise what her/his patients are doing, and analyse patients' progression in a particular routine.

About the challenge games, these also address cognitive stimulation. We are integrating several games in this set since we want to address different everyday life scenarios in order to engage children that have different interests and preferences. We started by implementing "Eco" (Fig. 2), which refers to the recycling theme since it was easy to set up providing scenarios that could easily include the movements previously defined. "Noir" (Fig. 2) is another game that focuses on private detectives, in night environments, that collect objects from clues and store them in a safe.

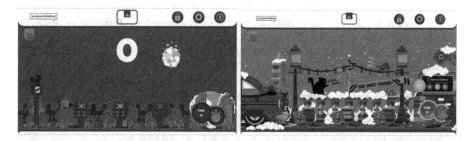

**Fig. 2.** Challenge games interfaces: "Eco, The Last Boy Scout" and "Noir, Cats Have 7 Lives".

In all games, the objects that must be caught appear only at points that will require the patient to perform the movements trained in the routines game. The games present several levels to the patient, based on different features, such as: with/without time limit; more or fewer objects to caught; objects can appear on predefined zones; only touch the objects, caught them or bring them to the bins/safes; among others. The patient can earn points and have a classification in a global ranking, among other functionalities related to each game. Therapists can configure the games towards each one of her/his patients, defining profiles that take into account that each child presents very particular characteristics. The way engagement with the games works with one child may differ greatly from another child.

Initially, a calibration process must be done taking into account the arms of the user. The objects will appear in points according to the calibration obtained in order to make the user perform the movements predefined by the therapist.

## 3   Conclusions and Future Work

This paper presented "just Physio kidding", which is focused on interactive and smart rehabilitation towards children with special needs, exploiting the Gamification and NUI concepts. The project aims to encourage physical exercise in order to stimulate cognition and combat physical deterioration, functioning as a complement to the work of therapists, with and without their live supervision. User tests with children and an acceptance evaluation with a physiotherapist were conducted in a clinic in order to align the development with the needs of the health professionals that lead with these "special patients". The results were very positive, and children were selected to integrate a participatory design process for the rest of the development. This process will be important to gather insights on how the games should be personalised towards the potential end-users of jPk.

**Acknowledgments.** We would like to thank physiotherapy clinic "Cresce com Amor", in Póvoa de Santa Iria, Portugal, for providing the support needed for the testings with the real end-users, which are the children. Moreover, we wish to thank therapist Ana Carolina Bernardo for using her expertise in the evaluation of jPk.

## References

1. Waddington, J., Linehan, C., Gerling, K., Hicks, K., Hodgson, T.L.: Participatory design of therapeutic video games for young people with neurological vision impairment. In: Proceedings of CHI 2015, pp. 3533–3542. ACM, New York (2015)
2. Deterding, S., Sicart, M., Nacke, L., O'Hara, K., Dixon, D.: Gamification: using game-design elements in non-gaming contexts. In: Proceedings of CHI 2011 Extended Abstracts on Human Factors in Computing Systems (CHI EA 2011), pp. 2425–2428. ACM, New York (2011)
3. Wiemeyer, J., Kliem, A.: Serious games in prevention and rehabilitation - a new panacea for elderly people? Eur. Rev. Aging Phys. Activity **9**(1), 41–50 (2012)

4. Kato, P.M., Cole, S.W., Bradlyn, A.S., Pollock, B.H.: A video game improves behavioral outcomes in adolescents and young adults with cancer: a randomized trial. Pediatrics **122**(2), 305–317 (2008)
5. Achtman, R.L., Green, C.S., Bavelier, D.: Video games as a tool to train visual skills. Restor. Neurol. Neurosci. **26**(4–5), 435–446 (2008)
6. Hernandez, H.A., Graham, T.C.N., Fehlings, D., Switzer, L., Ye, Z., Bellay, Q., Hamza, M. A., Savery, C., Stach, T.: Design of an exergaming station for children with cerebral palsy. In: Proceedings of CHI 2012, pp. 2619–2628. ACM, New York (2012)
7. Chang, C.-Y., Lange, B., Zhang, M., Koenig, S., Requejo, P., Somboon, N., Sawchuk, A.A., Rizzo, A.A.: Towards pervasive physical rehabilitation using Microsoft Kinect. In: Proceedings of PervasiveHealth 2012, pp. 159–162. ICST, Brussels (2012)
8. Clark, R.A., Pua, Y.-H., Bryant, A.L., Hunt, M.A.: Validity of the Microsoft Kinect for providing lateral trunk lean feedback during gait retraining. Gait Posture **38**(4), 1064–1066 (2013)
9. Madeira, R.N., Costa, L., Postolache, O.: PhysioMate - pervasive physical rehabilitation based on NUI and gamification. In: Proceedings of EPE 2014, pp. 612–616. IEEE (2014)
10. Rosenbaum, P., Paneth, N., Leviton, A., Goldstein, M., Bax, M., Damiano, D., Dan, B., Jacobsson, B.: A report: the definition and classification of cerebral palsy April 2006. Dev. Med. Child Neurol. Suppl. **109**, 8–14 (2007)
11. Hamari, J., Koivisto, J., Sarsa, H.: Does gamification work? – A literature review of empirical studies on gamification. In: Proceedings of System Sciences 2014, pp. 3025–3034. IEEE (2014)

# An Innovative Virtual Reality-Based Training Program for the Rehabilitation of Cognitive Frail Patients

Elisa Pedroli[1]([⊠]), Silvia Serino[1,2], Marco Stramba-Badiale[3], and Giuseppe Riva[1,2]

[1] Applied Technology for Neuro-Psychology Lab,
IRCCS Istituto Auxologico Italiano, Via Magnasco 2, 20149 Milan, Italy
{e.pedroli, s.serino}@auxologico.it,
giuseppe.riva@unicatt.it
[2] Psychology Department, Catholic University of Milan,
Largo Gemelli, 1, 20123 Milan, Italy
[3] Department of Geriatrics and Cardiovascular Medicine,
IRCCS Istituto Auxologico Italiano, Via Mosè Bianchi, 20149 Milan, Italy
stramba_badiale@auxologico.it

**Abstract.** Cognitive Frailty is one of the most common age-related disabilities in elderly. The two most damage cognitive domain in these patients are memory and executive functions. An innovative virtual reality-based training program for the rehabilitation of cognitive frail patients are proposed. The training is focused both on memory and executive functions and is possible to combine the two tasks according to the needs of the patients. The program could be done both with low-end (personal computer) and high-end (CAVE) virtual reality systems to guarantee the continuity of treatment from the hospital to home.

**Keywords:** Cognitive rehabilitation · Memory · Executive functions
Virtual reality · CAVE

## 1 Introduction

### 1.1 Cognitive Deficit in Elderly

Cognitive impairment in the elderly is one of the most common age-related disabilities and, to prevent the negative consequences of this decline, it is usually accepted how it is important to act promptly by targeting rehabilitation programs. Accordingly, the focus of intervention should be in the pre-clinical or early stage of the cognitive impairment. Prompt interventions could improve the ability of the elderly individuals and preserve their autonomy, thus avoiding an early hospitalization.

Recently, the International Consensus Group composed of the International Academy on Nutrition and Aging (IANA) and the International Association of Gerontology and Geriatrics (IAGG) [1] proposed the identification of the Cognitive Frailty (CF) to better describe elderly individuals who are at a preclinical stage.

© ICST Institute for Computer Sciences, Social Informatics and Telecommunications Engineering 2018
N. Oliver et al. (Eds.): MindCare 2016/Fabulous 2016/IIoT 2015, LNICST 207, pp. 62–66, 2018.
https://doi.org/10.1007/978-3-319-74935-8_8

The two main criteria was used to correctly recognize this syndrome:

- the presence of cognitive impairment and physical frailty;
- the exclusion of any other types of dementia.

Physical Frailty could be diagnosed when patients show at least 3 of these 5 physical criteria: (1) slow gait speed, (2) unintentional weight loss, (3) weak muscle strength, (4) exhaustion, and (5) sedentary behavior [2].

However, there are no clear indications about battery for the assessment of CF. Understanding the unique cognitive profile of patients with CF could lead to a prompt diagnosis and a timely rehabilitative intervention which is crucial for the potential reversibility and prevention of CF [1–3].

Delrieu and colleagues [3] have made a first attempt to define a neuropsychological profile of patients with CF. Specifically, they found deficits in processing speed, selective attention, free recall, and mental flexibility. Impairment in Executive Functions (EF) is the most common outcome of studies about the neuropsychological profile of CF [3–5].

Beside impairments in EF, another common deficit in elderly individuals may be found in a very specific domain: Spatial Memory (SM). Specifically, topographical disorientation is one of the most common deficits in the early stage of dementia, especially in Alzheimer Disease (AD) [6–8]. A recent study indicated that long-term allocentric representation may become inaccessible for a successful retrieval in patients with AD.

Both EF and SM deficits are complex phenomena that the classical assessment and rehabilitation protocols are not able to detect and manage adequately. A more ecological and customized procedure could help clinicians to improve the quality of the clinical practice.

## 1.2 Virtual Reality and Neurorehabilitation

Virtual Reality (VR) is a useful technology for neurorehabilitation, thanks to its peculiar characteristics. Using a virtual environments for the assessment and rehabilitation allows to increase the ecological validity and to control and manipulate the tasks according to the needs of patients, to adapt the difficulty levels of a task, and to engage patients in their training [9]. Moreover, by using VR, it is possible to drive and control the patients' performances in a functional, purposeful and motivating way, specifically for the rehabilitation protocols [10].

Specifically, for the treatment of EF, the goal is to create a task that allows patients to deal with every-day life situations. These situations require a more complex series of abilities compared to classic protocols: patients have concrete goals to achieve and a high degree of cognitive flexibility is required to elaborate different strategies to solve the problems and to inhibit inappropriate behaviors [11].

Moreover, VR is a useful tool to analyze impairment in the ability to manage spatial representations. Thanks to this technology, the therapist can induces interference in the egocentric representation and forces the use of long-term allocentric representation using a strategy known as "virtual disorientation," [12].

In summary, VR is an important technology for the improvement and amelioration of the classical paper and pencil protocol used in clinical settings. In the last decade, VR-based protocols have been developed for many neurological diseases, for both motor [13] and cognitive [14] impairments.

## 2   Virtual Rehabilitation Protocols

### 2.1   Cognitive Stimulations for the Elderly

Here, we present two different highly-ecological virtual rehabilitation protocols for EF and SM developed specifically for frail patients. Both protocols could be implemented using low-end and high-end virtual reality systems.

#### 2.1.1   Executive Functions

In order to stimulate the executive functions, we developed a VR-based training in a virtual supermarket. The protocol is based on the Virtual Multiple Errands Test (VMET), a VR-based assessment for the EF developed by Riva and colleagues [11, 15], itself inspired by the Multiple Errands Test (MET) [16, 17]. During the task, patients are able to move around in the supermarket and they are requested to select several products on shelves following precise rules. For the VR-based rehabilitation protocol, 10 different tasks with increasing difficulty are developed. Each task has different rules and different goals and may require a different aspect of the executive function domain to be solved. At the beginning of each session, the patient and the clinician analyze the task and the rules in order to understand and plan the different steps needed to solve the task. The clinician helps the patient during all the tasks in order to avoid the main errors and, at the end of the task, conducts a brief discussion about the outcome of the task. The software automatically records every object taken from the shelves and the path taken by the patient.

#### 2.1.2   Spatial Memory

In the virtual city developed for the training, patients can move around with a common joypad. As in the protocol for the rehabilitation of EF, 10 different tasks are created for the rehabilitation of SM. Each task is divided in two phases: encoding and retrieval. In the encoding phase, patients are asked to search for one, two or three objects located in some predefined place in the city. In this first phase, the exploration always starts from the center of the city.

In the retrieval part, patients are asked to remember and reach the place where the objects were located before. Here, the starting point is different for each session and is one of the cardinal points where the patient does not return.

Between the two phases of the first five tasks, the clinician shows an allocentric map of the city and shows the patient the starting point of the retrieval phase in order to simplify the use of allocentric representation.

If the patient has problems in remembering the target point, the software provides a cue, a green path that connects the present position of the subject to the forgotten point. The software automatically records the path taken by the patient, when all target points have been achieved, and if the cue has been used. This task is developed accordingly with the "Mental Frame Syncing" theory [9].

Before the rehabilitation training patient underwent to a complete neuropsychological and physical assessment in order to evaluate the CF. Only eligible patients are selected and started with the rehabilitation program.

Accordingly with the cognitive profile every sessions could include one or both protocols. After the 10 sessions a new cognitive assessment were done.

## 3   Discussion

Both the proposed protocols for cognitive rehabilitation are in the test phase with low-end and high-end virtual reality systems. The preliminary results are very encouraging and convince us to continue with the experiment.

An important aspect of neurorehabilitation that will be implemented in our innovative system is motor rehabilitation, because several studies show the efficacy of the virtual rehabilitation programs for many physical impairments [13]. Balance and prevention of falls are two main aspects of the therapeutic plan for frailty patients on which to focus attention [18]. Both of these goals are easily manageable within the CAVE system, but the development of new protocols is still in progress.

Thanks to this advanced technology, the possibility exists to create complex and integrated protocols to maximize the efficacy of the treatment plan. An increasing number of studies showed that the effectiveness of a treatment that combines the cognitive and motor aspects [19, 20].

Another important aspect is the assessment of both cognitive and motor deficits. VR is an important tool because it allows ecological and standardized environments for a more precise and valid assessment. Many studies have analyzed the use of VR-based assessment protocols for cognitive impairment with very positive results [14, 15]. Clearly, a more precise assessment method allows an early diagnosis and a prompt rehabilitation treatment aimed at increasing the autonomy and the health of frail patients.

**Acknowledgments.** This work was supported by the Italian funded project "High-end and Low-End Virtual Reality Systems for the Rehabilitation of Frailty in the Elderly" -PE-2013-02355948.

## References

1. Kelaiditi, E., et al.: Cognitive frailty: rational and definition from an (IANA/IAGG) international consensus group. J. Nutr. Health Aging **17**(9), 726–734 (2013)
2. Fried, L.P., et al.: Frailty in older adults evidence for a phenotype. J. Gerontol. Ser. A Biol. Sci. Med. Sci. **56**(3), M146–M157 (2001)
3. Delrieu, J., et al.: Neuropsychological profile of "cognitive frailty" subjects in MAPT study. J. Prevent. Alzheimer's Dis. **3**(3), 151 (2016)
4. Montero-Odasso, M.M., et al.: Disentangling cognitive-frailty: results from the gait and brain study. J. Gerontol. Ser. A Biol. Sci. Med. Sci. (2016). glw044

5. Shimada, H., et al.: Impact of cognitive frailty on daily activities in older persons. J. Nutr. Health Aging, pp. 1–7
6. Iachini, T., et al.: Visuospatial memory in healthy elderly, AD and MCI: a review. Curr. Aging Sci. **2**(1), 43–59 (2009)
7. Guariglia, C.C., Nitrini, R.: Topographical disorientation in Alzheimer's disease. Arq. Neuropsiquiatr. **67**(4), 967–972 (2009)
8. Aguirre, G.K., D'Esposito, M.: Topographical disorientation: a synthesis and taxonomy. Brain **122**(9), 1613–1628 (1999)
9. Riva, G., Gaggioli, A.: Rehabilitation as empowerment: the role of advanced technologies. In: Gaggioli, A., et al. (eds.) Advanced Technologies in Rehabilitation - Empowering Cognitive, Physical, Social and Communicative Skills Through Virtual Reality, Robots, Wearable Systems and Brain-Computer Interfaces, pp. 3–22. IOS Press, Amsterdam (2009)
10. Bohil, C.J., Alicea, B., Biocca, F.A.: Virtual reality in neuroscience research and therapy. Nat. Rev. Neurosci. **12**(12), 752–762 (2011)
11. Raspelli, S., et al.: Validation of a Neuro Virtual Reality-based version of the Multiple Errands Test for the assessment of executive functions. Stud. Health Technol. Inform. **167**, 92–97 (2011)
12. Bosco, A., et al.: Assessing human reorientation ability inside virtual reality environments: the effects of retention interval and landmark characteristics. Cogn. Process. **9**(4), 299–309 (2008)
13. Mirelman, A., et al.: Addition of a non-immersive virtual reality component to treadmill training to reduce fall risk in older adults (V-TIME): a randomised controlled trial. Lancet **388**, 1170–1182 (2016)
14. Pedroli, E., et al.: Assessment and rehabilitation of neglect using virtual reality: a systematic review. Front. Behav. Neurosci. **9** (2015)
15. Cipresso, P., et al.: Virtual multiple errands test (VMET): a virtual reality- based tool to detect early executive functions deficit in Parkinson's disease. Front. Behav. Neurosci. **8** (2014)
16. Alderman, N., et al.: Ecological validity of a simplified version of the multiple errands shopping test. J. Int. Neuropsychol. Soc. **9**(01), 31–44 (2003)
17. Shallice, T., Burgess, P.W.: Deficits in strategy application following frontal lobe damage in man. Brain **114**(2), 727–741 (1991)
18. de Labra, C., et al.: Effects of physical exercise interventions in frail older adults: a systematic review of randomized controlled trials. BMC Geriatr. **15**(1), 1 (2015)
19. Wang, X., et al.: Cognitive motor interference for preventing falls in older adults: a systematic review and meta-analysis of randomised controlled trials. Age Ageing **44**(2), 205–212 (2015)
20. Schoene, D., et al.: The effect of interactive cognitive-motor training in reducing fall risk in older people: a systematic review. BMC Geriatr. **14**(1), 1 (2014)

# COLLEGO: An Interactive Platform for Studying Joint Action During an Ecological Collaboration Task

Alice Chirico[1]([✉]), Serena Graziosi[2], Francesco Ferrise[2],
Alberto Gallace[3], Cedric Mosconi[4], Marie Jasmine Cazzaniga[4],
Valentino Zurloni[5,6], Massimiliano Elia[5], Francesco Cerritelli[7,8,9],
Fabrizia Mantovani[5,6], Alessandro D'Ausilio[10], Pietro Cipresso[1,11],
Giuseppe Riva[1,11], and Andrea Gaggioli[1,11]

[1] Department of Psychology, Università Cattolica del Sacro Cuore, Milan, Italy
{alice.chirco,pietro.cipresso,giuseppe.riva,
andrea.gaggioli}@unicatt.it
[2] Department of Mechanical Engineering, Politecnico di Milano, Milan, Italy
{serena.graziosi,francesco.ferrise}@polimi.it
[3] Department of Psychology and Milan Centre for Neuroscience,
University of Milano Bicocca, Milan, Italy
alberto.gallacel@unimib.it
[4] Department of Psychology, University of Milano Bicocca, Milan, Italy
{c.mosconi3,m.cazzaniga24}@campus.unimib.it
[5] Department of Human Sciences for Education "Riccardo Massa",
University of Milano-Bicocca, Milan, Italy
{valentino.zurloni,fabrizia.mantovani}@unimib.it,
m.elia5@campus.unimib.it
[6] CESCOM (Center for Studies in Communication Sciences),
University of Milano-Bicocca, Milan, Italy
[7] Clinical-Based Human Research Department,
Centre for Osteopathic Medicine Collaboration, Pescara, Italy
francesco.cerritelli@gmail.com
[8] Department of Neuroscience, Imaging and Clinical Sciences,
"G. D'Annunzio" University of Chieti-Pescara, Pescara, Italy
[9] ITAB-Institute for Advanced Biomedical Technologies, "G. D'Annunzio"
University of Chieti-Pescara, Pescara, Italy
[10] Center of Translational Neurophysiology,
IIT - Istituto Italiano di Tecnologia - CTNSC@UniFe, Ferrara, Italy
alessandro.dausilio@iit.it
[11] IRCCS Istituto Auxologico Italiano, Milan, Italy
{p.cipresso,g.riva,a.gaggioli}@auxologico.it

**Abstract.** We describe the implementation and preliminary validation of an interactive platform – COLLEGO – to investigate joint action in a goal-oriented collaborative task. The platform records the interaction sequence of two partners alternating their leader/follower role. Two sensitized wooden surfaces are placed in front of each participant, who can use 6 cubes to build the tower. Any time a cube is picked/released, time stamp (ms) and position of selected objects are

© ICST Institute for Computer Sciences, Social Informatics and Telecommunications Engineering 2018
N. Oliver et al. (Eds.): MindCare 2016/Fabulous 2016/IIoT 2015, LNICST 207, pp. 67–72, 2018.
https://doi.org/10.1007/978-3-319-74935-8_9

recorded. A case study showing how data are collected and analyzed to study dyad performance during the task is described. Finally, potential applications of the proposed solution are discussed.

**Keywords:** Human-human interaction · Joint action · Synchronization Performance · Time-series analysis · Sensors

# 1  Introduction

Humans are social animals and as such, they are able to work together co-operatively in order accomplish a shared goal [1]. This is a crucial ability to survive and it is regarded as "joint-action", more widely defined as "*any form of social interaction whereby two or more individuals coordinate their actions in space and time to bring about a change in the environment*" [2].

The experimental study of joint action has been oriented towards the investigation of simplified forms of human interaction, in order to exert experimental control over the parameters affecting behavior and motor executions [3]. Nevertheless, coordinating with another human in everyday life entails a continuous information flow exchange that needs to be experimentally reproduced in ecologically valid ways. On other hand, constraints characterizing an experimental setting do not help pursuing this goal. To address this issue, D'Ausilio et al. introduced and validated [4] the "tower-building task", a goal-directed ecological task to investigate continuous interaction in joint action (see Fig. 1).

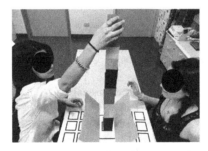

**Fig. 1.** An example of the "tower-building task" described in [4] to study continuous interaction in joint action.

The task can be used to study motor coordination in relation to several cognitive abilities. It could be also applied for rehabilitation or training purposes. Moreover, it may be used to facilitate the process of planning complex actions that can be grouped in super-ordinate categories as action strategies. Finally, the task is intuitive, minimally invasive, and allows for a continuous interaction among partners.

Given the potentials of this tower-building task, the aim of the present project was to build a sensorized platform to automatically log and record participants' interactions, to investigate joint action in an experimentally-controlled but also ecologically-valid way. The key design requirements were as follows:

- Automatic data collection: the platform had to be able to assess main collaborative interaction parameters automatically (namely, cube position, time reaction for the rising of each cube).
- Continuous recording of building dynamic: platform had to be able to record the sequence of cubes, which were selected by the two partners.
- Modular and flexible design: platform had to be composed of different basic operative modules, which can be eventually integrated with other computational modules/interfaces or other assessment instruments (e.g. physiological sensors).
- Open source hardware and software: platform had to be affordable and easy to build/modify/adapt according to users' needs.

## 2 Technical Setup

Following the procedure of the tower-building task described in [4], two participants are asked to seat one in front of each other. One participant acts as leader, and the other as follower. The leader has to pick a cube from the platform and to start building the tower. The follower has to imitate the leader, thus take a cube of the same color and put on top of the previous one, until the tower is completed. At the beginning of the experiment each participant is provided with six cubes placed in front of him. The cubes are colored in: green, light and dark brown. Each cube (the length of the edge is 60 mm) is made of wood and weights approximately 160 g. The distance between two adjacent cubes is 40 mm. The main dimensions of the rectangle containing the cubes are $272 \times 172$ mm. Both platforms are obtained from a 3 mm thick wooden sheet.

Each platform is equipped with six push buttons, which detect whether the cube has been positioned over the platform, or lifted up. Each button is positioned in a 6 mm square hole under the cube and is plugged to a digital pin of an Arduino UNO board (www.arduino.cc). The initial state of each button is "pushed". Every time a state change of the button is detected (i.e. a cube has been moved away from the platform, or put back on it), Arduino sends a string to a pc through a standard serial communication (baud rate 115200) containing: the timestamp (in ms), the name of the button and the state. These signals are acquired by a software developed in Processing (https:// processing.org) which displays, in real-time, the state of the platform to the experimenter. Data are automatically saved in a text file. At the beginning of each experiment all buttons, of the two platforms, are in the "pushed" condition with the cube placed over them. Then, as the experiment continues, the number of pushed buttons diminishes, theoretically, with a step of one button per platform and per task. However, this not always occurs and a post-processing phase is necessary to clean data. To this aim, two more applications have been developed.

One application (developed in Processing) takes as input the text file and creates a movie reproducing what the experimenter has seen during the experiment (see Fig. 2). The other, developed in MATLAB (www.mathworks.com), takes at once all the text files of the trials and clean the data from noise generated during the experiment. Examples of noise are the following: during an experiment the subject can hit a cube while is picking another one, or he can hesitate while lifting one. An algorithm, which keeps the last time the cube has been lifted, has been developed to filter the data. These results are compared with the notes taken by the experimenter, who is asked to keep track of the errors happened during each trial, the failure of the trial and so on. Finally, the post-processing software analyses all the ten trials of a couple and gives as output a unique matrix containing the timestamp and the position of all the cubes that have been lifted from the platform. The timestamp now is computed with respect to the first cube that has been lifted, in order to allow a comparison among all the subjects. This matrix is exported into an Excel sheet for further statistical analysis, to be run in IBM SPSS. Compared to the use of a tracking system, the designed system has two main advantages. First, it is a low-cost, portable and open-source solution representing an optimum trade-off between data accuracy and the complexity of the technology used. This has been possible shifting the focus of the experiment from the kinematic of the subjects' movements to the output/consequences of their actions. This aspect introduces the second advantage which is related to easiness of data elaboration. Indeed, while the tracking system provides, as output, the whole trajectory of the hand, the platform is focused on automatically extrapolating the data of real interest which is the moment when the cube is released.

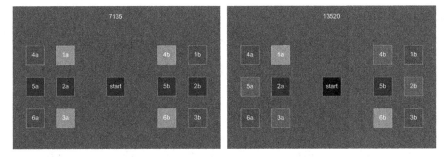

**Fig. 2.** This application allows the experimenter to replay each trial. The images represent two different frames of a trial (7135 ms and 13520 ms). (Color figure online)

## 3   Case Study

We tested the platform with 24 female couples (mean age = 22, 33; S.D. = 2, 155) and 24 male couples (mean age = 23, 38; S.D. = 2, 712), all right-handed. The overall 48 couples executed the tower-building task during 10 consecutive trials. They were required to build the tower using only one hand, and positioning a cube at time.

Figure 3 illustrates the variations of dyad performance (time taken to complete trials) of the whole sample across the 10 trials. As expected, linear reduction in execution time across trials may suggest improvement in group performance. These findings suggest that the measures taken by the platform are able to capture learning performance dynamics (Fig. 3).

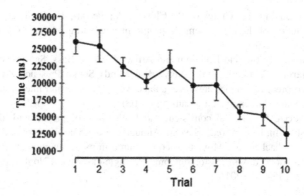

**Fig. 3.** Descriptive plot for the 48 couples indicating the average duration per each trial execution during the task.

## 4   Discussion and Conclusion

We described an interactive platform for investigating joint action in an ecologically-valid way. The task does not require any training, is short enough to maintain high levels of engagement, and captures performance data with minimally-invasive recording. This goal-oriented, game-like scenario is based on open source hardware and software components, in order to ensure easy reproducibility and low-cost setup. Findings of the pilot validation study showed that the platform is able to accurately and reliably measure performance of interacting participants. This suggests the potential usefulness of the proposed solution for joint action research. In particular, the engaging and motivating characteristics of the tower-building task could be exploited to study motor coordination in relation to subjective dimensions of partners' collaborative experience, such as the experience of "flow" [5] and social presence (i.e. feelings of mental connectedness [6, 7]. Finally, a more speculative application of this tool might be any doctor-patient relationship, since there is some evidence regarding the potential relevance of movement synchronization in psychotherapy [8].

## References

1. Visco-Comandini, F., Ferrari-Toniolo, S., Satta, E., Papazachariadis, O., Gupta, R., Nalbant, L.E., Battaglia-Mayer, A.: Do non-human primates cooperate? Evidences of motor coordination during a joint action task in macaque monkeys. Cereb. Cortex **70**, 115–127 (2015)
2. Sebanz, N., Bekkering, H., Knoblich, G.: Joint action: bodies and minds moving together. Trends. Cogn. Sci. **10**(2), 70–76 (2006)
3. D'Ausilio, A., Novembre, G., Fadiga, L., Keller, P.E.: What can music tell us about social interaction? Trends Cogn. Sci. **19**(3), 111–114 (2015)

4. D'Ausilio, A., Badino, L., Cipresso, P., Chirico, A., Ferrari, E., Riva, G., Gaggioli, A.: Automatic imitation of the arm kinematic profile in interacting partners. Cogn. Process. **16** (Supp 1), 197–201 (2015)
5. Csikszentmihalyi, M.: Beyond Boredom and Anxiety. Jossey-Bass, San Francisco (2000)
6. Biocca, F., Harms, C.: Guide to the Networked Minds Social Presence Inventory v. 1.2: Measures of co-presence, social presence, subjective symmetry, and intersubjective symmetry. Michigan State University, East Lansing (2003)
7. Harms, C., Biocca, F.: Internal consistency and reliability of the networked minds social presence measure. In: Rey, A. (ed.) Seventh Annual International Workshop, Presence (2004)
8. Ramseyer, F., Tschacher, W.: Movement coordination in psychotherapy: synchrony of hand movements is associated with session outcome. A single-case study. Nonlinear Dyn. Psychol. Life Sci. **20**(2), 145–166 (2016)

# Non-pharmacological Approaches
# in the Depression Treatment - Strengths
# and Weaknesses of Mobile Applications Use

Petra Maresova[(✉)] and Blanka Klimova

University of Hradec Kralove, Rokitanskeho 62,
50003 Hradec Kralove, Czech Republic
{Petra.maresova,blanka.klimova}@uhk.cz

**Abstract.** As the prevalence of mental illnesses such as depression and anxiety continues to grow, clinicians have turned to mobile applications as tools for aiding and supporting their patients' treatment. These applications can be especially helpful for teenagers and young adults suffering from mental illness due to their frequent use of technology as a means of communication. Depression is the fourth frequent cause of death. It can affect almost anybody, including children. In most cases non-pharmacological treatment is preferred since it is less invasive, has fewer side-effects and sometimes it is also less expensive. The paper aims to explore the effectiveness of the use of mobile applications, which is demonstrated clinically and consequently, the focus is also put on the criteria evaluating the quality, strengths and weaknesses of current mobile health applications. The results show that clinical trials confirm some positive effects of mobile applications, however the evidence is rather low and further monitoring is needed.

**Keywords:** Health · Mobile applications · Depression · Treatment

## 1 Introduction

At present mental disorders affect approximately 450 million people around the world [1]. Depression disorder is probably the most serious one. Nowadays, depression as a type of chronic disease represents a global threat and burdens economic and social systems of both individuals and governments worldwide [2–4]. This concerns also the costs on pharmacological and non-pharmacological treatment. Nevertheless, in most cases non-pharmacological treatment is preferred since it is less invasive, has fewer side-effects and sometimes it is also less expensive. One of these non-pharmacological approaches is the so-called mHealth (mobile health); the use of mobile devices for the practice of medicine and public health.

According to the World Health Organization report [5], mHealth is a globally adopted technology. Employers, too, recognise that facilitating employees' health maintenance is advantageous and reported successful trials for mental health issues. In addition, many current m-health initiatives focus on outdated, unidirectional models of patient communication (e.g., exclusively collecting data, providing information or

© ICST Institute for Computer Sciences, Social Informatics and Telecommunications Engineering 2018
N. Oliver et al. (Eds.): MindCare 2016/Fabulous 2016/IIoT 2015, LNICST 207, pp. 73–77, 2018.
https://doi.org/10.1007/978-3-319-74935-8_10

sending reminders) [5]. The use of mobile technologies, in particular, is rapidly evolving within the field of tele-mental health. mHealth is conducted on "mobile phones, patient monitoring devices, personal digital assistants (PDAs), and other wireless devices" [6].

The purpose of this article is to explore the most recent randomized controlled clinical trial studies which prove efficacy of the use of mobile applications in the diagnostics or treatment of depression. Consequently, the focus is also put on the criteria evaluating the quality, strengths and weaknesses of current mobile health applications. In conclusion, the authors list the main strengths and weaknesses of mobile applications in the diagnosis and treatment of depression.

## 2   Methods

The methods used in this study include a method of literature search of the studies focused on the impacts of individual applications for people with depression and on the specification of criteria evaluating quality of these applications. After removing redundancies, abstracts were analyzed by two research workers and other irrelevant articles were excluded from the content point of view. Eventually, 11 full-text research studies were analyzed. Since technologies develop fast and not all the applications for patients with depression are specified in research studies, other Internet sources were used.

## 3   Use of Mobile Applications in the Treatment of Depression

As the prevalence of mental illnesses such as depression and anxiety continues to grow, clinicians have turned to mobile applications as tools for aiding and supporting their patients' treatment. These applications can be especially helpful for teenagers and young adults suffering from mental illness due to their frequent use of technology as a means of communication. Health applications for depression – criteria of effectiveness However, it is very crucial to choose the right ones, which can meet certain criteria. According to [7], mHealth applications must be safe, accurate, effective, secure, and protect privacy to be used by patients, recommended by health care professionals, and eventually reimbursed [8].

In the study by [7] these criteria were discussed in a more detail and the applications assessed according to three measures of effectiveness: perceived effectiveness, research evidence base for an app, and whether or not the app claimed that the effectiveness was tested [8]. The key criteria with respect to depressions seem to be as follows: password protection, number of consumer ratings, explicit privacy policy.

Another criteria also include: interactiveness/feedback, encryption, basis of research, software support, import/export capabilities, developer contactable, personalization, specificity of intervention, source of funding for research, discloses potential risks, effectiveness (perceived), continuous availability of data, effectiveness tested (claimed by app), ease of use, advertising policy stated and errors and performance issues [7, 8].

According to [9], the smartphones should support built-in Bluetooth HDP for standard Bluetooth communication with medical devices. This will enable the smartphone applications to work with medical devices from different vendors. Other technical specifications which appear to be quite important are: long battery life, sufficiently large screen size, fast data input, virus-free computer, no magnetic interference with medical devices, efficient patient-physician interactions, avoidance of loss or theft, and data privacy and security [9].

The privacy and security concerns of storing or communicating patient data with smartphones should be addressed cautiously. These security features of smartphones, while not available for all devices, may be useful: data backup, encryption of stored patient data, remote wiping to destroy all data on a device in case of loss or theft, and securely encrypted wireless data transmission over WiFi [10–12] applications.

Finally, personal data must be considered when using the mobile applications, which is also closely connected with the rules of handling these data. In many ways, these areas are not still legally specified. According to [13], when using an application, the following criteria must be specified: compliance with privacy (user should be informed how or for how long his/her data are stored), security (protection against viruses), accuracy of content, safety (the app provides information on the proper way of using it. It warns the user against possible health dangers (side effects) related to the use of the app for different purposes or without following the suggested protocol).

Figure 1 below illustrates the principal criteria of applications quality for the treatment of depression discussed in most of the research studies.

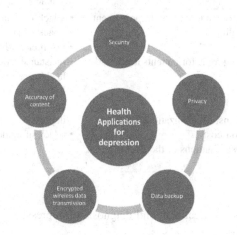

**Fig. 1.** Criteria of applications quality for the treatment of depression

## 4   Discussion and Conclusion

The number of mobile health applications is rapidly growing thanks to the rapid development of these technologies worldwide. As far as the treatment and diagnosis of depression disorders are concerned, there is a general support for their use [14]. Since it is quite a new field of research, more clinical trials are needed to prove efficacy of mobile health applications for the treatment and diagnosis of depression. This is in fact questioned in many studies, e.g., [15]. As Andersson and Titov [16] state, the Internet based programs supported by an experienced therapist can monitor and support patients before a crisis starts to develop. However, these interventions must be of good quality and sufficiently stimulating to engage patients with depression. In addition, their privacy data should be protected.

Generally, more promotion of the benefits of mobile health applications for the treatment and diagnosis of depression is needed. East and Harvard [17] propose several ways of improving this:

- raise awareness of evidence-based applications;
- infuse mental health mobile applications into graduate counsellor education;
- disseminate information about mobile health applications during clinical staff meetings;
- integrate mobile health applications into therapy; and
- publish research in this filed and present it at conferences.

Table 1 below summarizes the main strengths and weaknesses of using mobile

**Table 1.** The main strengths and weaknesses of using mobile health applications for the treatment and diagnosis of depression

| Strength | Weaknesses |
|---|---|
| • clinical trials show promising results; improvement of treatment accessibility; <br>• patient empowerment; <br>• efficient self-monitoring tools for patients in the early stages of the disease; <br>• suitable supporting therapies; <br>• cost-effectiveness; <br>• reduction of hospital institutionalization and care; <br>• lowering of prevention costs; <br>• reduction of visits, examinations at the doctor; <br>• cut of labor costs | • a lack of data security; <br>• a lack of standards; <br>• insufficient data backup; <br>• resistance from traditional healthcare providers; <br>• low awareness of benefits mobile applications for the treatment of depression; <br>• a lack of evidence-based programs |

health applications for the treatment and diagnosis of depression.

**Acknowledgement.** The paper was written with the support of the specific project grant "Economics and Managerial aspects in Biomedicine" granted by the University of Hradec Kralove, Czech Republic.

# References

1. mHealth Alliance. mHealth solutions for improving mental health and illnesses in the aging process, White Paper Series on mHealth and Aging (2013). http://www.mhealthknowledge. org/sites/default/files/7_mHA-Aging-Paper3_092713.pdf
2. Lönnqvist, J.: Major psychiatric disorders in suicide and suicide attempters. In: Wasserman, D., Wasserman, C. (eds.) Oxford Textbook of Suicidology and Suicide Prevention: A Global Approach, pp. 275–286. Oxford University Press, Oxford (2009)
3. Klimova, B., Maresova, P., Valis, M., Hort, J., Kuca, K.: Alzheimer's disease and language impairments: social intervention and medical treatment. Clin. Interv. Aging **10**, 1401–1408 (2015)
4. Maresova, P., Mohelska, H., Dolejs, J., Kuca, K.: Socio-economic aspects of Alzheimer's disease. Curr. Alzheimer Res. **12**(9), 903–911 (2015)
5. Evans, W.D., Abroms, L.C., Poropatich, R., Nielsen, P.E., Wallace, J.L.: Mobile health evaluation methods: the Text4baby case study. J. Health Commun. **17**(1), 22–29 (2012)
6. Kohn, R., Saxena, S., Levav, I., Saraceno, B.: The treatment gap in mental health care. Bull. World Health Organ. **82**(11), 858–866 (2004)
7. Powell, A.C., Torous, J., Chan, S., Raynor, G.S., Shwarts, E., Shanahan, M., Landman, A. B.: Interrater reliability of mHealth app rating measures: analysis of top depression and smoking cessation apps. JMIR **4**(1), e15 (2016)
8. Powell, A.C., Landman, A.B., Bates, D.W.: In search of a few good apps. JAMA **311**(18), 1851–1852 (2014)
9. Haller, G., Haller, D.M., Courvoisier, D.S., Lovis, C.: Handheld vs. laptop computers for electronic data collection in clinical research: a crossover randomized trial. J. Am. Med. Informatics Assoc. **16**, 651 (2009)
10. iPhone in Business. Security Overview (2016). http://images.apple.com/iphone/business/ docs/iPhone_Security.pdf
11. Palm webOS Security Overview for Enterprise (2016). http://www.hpwebos.com/us/assets/ pdfs/business/Palm_WhitePaper_Security.pdf
12. Device Administration (2016). http://developer.android.com/guide/topics/admin/device-admin.html
13. Ozdalga, E., Ozdalga, A., Ahuja, N.: The smarphone in Medicine: a review of current and potential use among physicians and students. J. Med. Internet Res. **14**(5), e128 (2012)
14. Hedman, E., Ljótsson, B., Lindefors, N.: Cognitive behavior therapy via the internet: a systematic review of applications, clinical efficacy and cost-effectiveness. Expert Rev. Pharmacoecon Outcomes Res. **12**, 745–764 (2012)
15. Ly, K.H., Janni, E., Wiede, R., Sedem, M., Donker, T., Carlberg, P., Andersson, G.: Experiences of a guided smart-based behavioral activation therapy for depression: a qualitative study. Internet Interv. **2**(1), 60–68 (2015)
16. Andersson, G., Titov, N.: Advantages and limitations of Internet-based interventions for common mental disorders. World Psychiatry **13**(1), 4–11 (2014)
17. East, M.L., Harvard, B.C.: Mental health mobile apps: from infusion to diffusion in the mental health social system. JMIR **2**(1), e10 (2015)

# FABULOUS 2016

# Assessment of Mechanical Stiffness of Jumping Using Force Plate

Nikola Mijailovic[1,2,3(✉)], Radivoje Radakovic[1,2,3],
Aleksandar Peulic[1,2,3], Neda Vidanovic[1,2,3], Djordje Dimitrijevic[1,2,3],
and Nenad Filipovic[1,2,3]

[1] Faculty of Engineering, University of Kragujevac,
Sestre Janjic 6, 34000 Kragujevac, Serbia
{nmijailovic, aleksandar.peulic, neda,
dimco, fica}@kg.ac.rs, dididisport@yahoo.com
[2] Bioengineering Research and Development Center (BioIRC),
Kragujevac, Serbia
[3] University of Kragujevac, Kragujevac, Serbia

**Abstract.** In this paper the basic information about methodology of assessment human body stiffness during vertical jump analysis is presented. Ten subjects (professional football player) perform ten periodic jumps and vertical ground reaction force is measured using a force plate with one axial load cell force sensor. The stiffness calculation is based on the analogy of the periodic jumping and oscillation movement of the system which consists of spring and body appropriate mass. The frequency of oscillation is obtained using Fourier transform.

**Keywords:** Vertical jump · Force plate · Mechanical stiffness

## 1 Introduction

Quantification and description of the of jumps performed during sports games, such as drop jump, squat jump, and counter movement jump is very important part of the measurement of the athletic performance in the sports. The standard method in jump analyzing is based on the use of a force sensors platform for ground reaction force measuring [1–3]. The force platform can measure force and torque during jump in different directions using a force sensor [4]. Improvement of electronic devices and gadgets in recent years has enabled us to measure jumping parameters by using wearable devices, such as sensors, in footwear [5]. This method gives much comfort and real conditions to subjects due to the fact that there is no bounded area for jumping performance. Simultaneously with force measuring, for complete biomechanical analyses it is also necessary to determine the position of a particular body part. For this purpose a high speed camera is used. The high speed camera records position marker points attached to the subject's leg, arm, hip, etc. with a frame rate of 100 Hz and higher. Using the software, 3D point coordinate of markers position can be reconstructed. It is necessary to use a number of cameras for this reconstruction. Alternatively, for position reconstruction different kinds of sensors, such as accelerometer [6], gyroscope,

© ICST Institute for Computer Sciences, Social Informatics and Telecommunications Engineering 2018
N. Oliver et al. (Eds.): MindCare 2016/Fabulous 2016/IIoT 2015, LNICST 207, pp. 81–86, 2018.
https://doi.org/10.1007/978-3-319-74935-8_11

goniometer and magnetometer [7] can be used. In this paper we presented a method for measuring force during jumping activity, using force plate platform and assessment of mechanical stiffness of human body. The mechanical stiffness play a very important role in assessment sportiest performance especially the tendency to the injuries.

## 2    Materials and Methods

The participants in experiments followed a standardized warming-up and stretching period. During the measurements, participants wore their own indoor sport shirts, shorts and sneakers. Participants were instructed to perform a number type of jumps: (squat jump, countermovement jump and hop). Their motion was recorded using two high speed cameras with a frame rate of 200 fps. The cameras with software for acquisition and image processing are part of Innovision Systems, Inc product for tracking motion with biomedical and sports application. Before performing jumping the system is calibrated.

The ground reaction force was sampled from the multi-axis AMTI force plate Fig. 1 at the rate of 300 Hz (© Advanced Mechanical Technology, Inc.). Before the start of the experiment, calibration was required to work out the space coordinate system of the field of view area. The calibration was performed fully in accordance with the manufacturer's instructions.

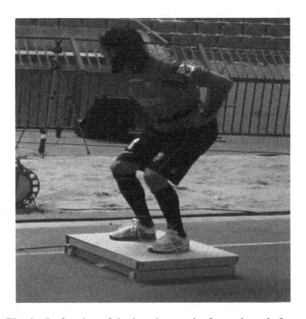

**Fig. 1.** Performing of the jumping on the force plate platform

The participants stood in front of the force plate. After the trigger was launched, each participant executed ten jumps one by one with their commonly period. Figure 2 shows signal of vertical force value during time for this type of jump.

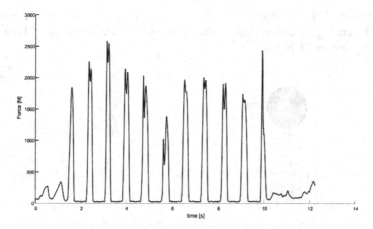

**Fig. 2.** Force signal during periodic jumps.

According to recorded signal the period of jumping is obtained. This is accomplished using the Fast Fourier transform FFT of the force signal.

On the Fig. 3 the amplitude of the Fourier transform is show what is known as amplitude characteristic of signal. The horizontal axis represents frequency of the signal and on the vertical axis is corresponding intensity of signal for that frequency. The peak with largest value is at point of zero frequency and it is mean value of signal. We considered only next peak at (1.2 Hz in case of this participant). This is actually the frequency of the jumping. Using this method by detecting second peak by range we can precisely obtained the jumping frequency during hop. The stiffness [N/m] of subject is given by relation

$$k_{jump} = (2\pi f)^2 m \qquad (1)$$

where $m$ is mass of the participant is experiment. The lower value of the mechanical stiffness points to the better performance of the sportiest and fewer penchant to the injuries.

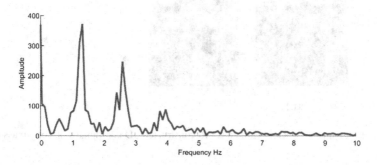

**Fig. 3.** Frequency spectra of the force signal

The relation between stiffness, body mass and frequency of periodic jumps is obtained by analogy between free oscillation of system which consist of body mass *m*and spring stiffness *k* Fig. 4.

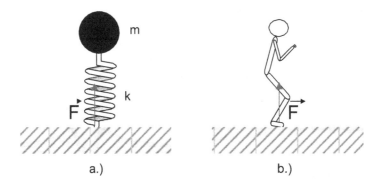

a.)                                    b.)

**Fig. 4.** Analogy between (a) spring oscillation and (b) periodic jumping

The frequency of spring oscillation is given by relation:

$$f = \frac{1}{2\pi}\sqrt{k/m} \tag{1}$$

where $k$ is corresponding spring stiffness. For jumping the analog stiffness can be defined and adopt that mass of performer jumping and frequency of jumping by the corresponding mass-spring system. The ground reaction force during jumping is analog with the straining force in the spring.

For the all performers the body center mass displacement is measured using innovision camera system Fig. 5.

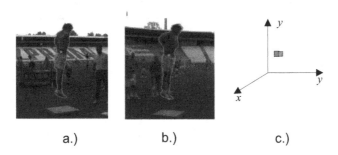

a.)                    b.)                    c.)

**Fig. 5.** (a) Left camera (b) Right camera (c) Reconstructed 3D coordinates of body mass center

The coordinates of body mass center are obtained by calculation momentum of contour of performer body during jumping.

## 3  Results

In the Table 1 the mechanical stiffness of body for ten subjects is shown. The stiffness is calculated using Eq. (1).

**Table 1.**  Body weight and stiffness for ten subjects

| Subject no. | Body weight [kg] | Stiffness [N/m] |
|---|---|---|
| 1 | 72.2 | 3.1835e+03 |
| 2 | 74.8 | 3.4151e+03 |
| 3 | 76.4 | 4.2512e+03 |
| 4 | 63.6 | 4.9135e+03 |
| 5 | 87.0 | 5.2573e+03 |
| 6 | 62.2 | 4.3482e+03 |
| 7 | 68.3 | 4.5653e+03 |
| 8 | 59.9 | 3.6217e+03 |
| 9 | 73.5 | 4.4198e+03 |
| 10 | 72.1 | 4.7214e+03 |

The ground reaction force is related with the mechanical stiffness by relation

$$F_{ground} = K_{jump} \cdot x \tag{2}$$

where $x$ is displacement of the body mass center. In the Table 2 the measured and calculated displacement of the body center mass is shown. The difference of calculated and measured displacement occurs due to uncertainty of the mechanical stiffness.

**Table 2.**  Center mass displacement for ten subjects

| Subject no. | Center mass displacement [m] (obtained) | Center mass displacement [m] (measured) |
|---|---|---|
| 1 | 0.79 | 0.93 |
| 2 | 0.58 | 0.97 |
| 3 | 0.64 | 0.88 |
| 4 | 0.73 | 0.91 |
| 5 | 0.67 | 0.95 |
| 6 | 0.81 | 0.93 |
| 7 | 0.65 | 0.64 |
| 8 | 0.56 | 0.65 |
| 9 | 0.78 | 0.86 |
| 10 | 0.63 | 0.75 |

## 4 Conclusion and Discussion

In this paper the result of measuring force during performing periodic jumps is shown. The force plate platform is one of the basic devices for biomechanical analysis. The achieved force signal is used for calculation mechanical stiffness of human body during jump. The first step is calculation mean frequency of the jump using Fourier analysis and finally the stiffness is obtained using relation of free osculation of the spring and loaded by the body corresponding mass. The ten subjects participate in the experiment and stiffness is calculated using their body mass weight. The mechanical stiffness can be used as parameter for assessment sportsman performance. The lower stiffness value indicate a less stress of lower limb during jumping. The mechanical stiffness can be used for calculation body mass center displacement according to relation between force and stiffness. The acquired results suggest difference between calculated displacements and measured using high speed camera. This is repercussion of the adapted model of the just one spring and frequency of the jumping and exemption of influence of the complex movement whole body during performing jumping. In the future work we will try to calculate mechanical stiffness using more complex model which will be include consider a number of harmonics in spectra of force signal.

**Acknowledgments.** This paper is part of project III41007, funded by the Ministry of Education, Science and Technological Development of the Republic of Serbia.

## References

1. Cross, R.: Standing, walking, running, and jumping on a force plate. Am. J. Phys. **67**(4), 304–309 (1999)
2. Filipovic, N., Vulovic, R., Peulic, A., Radakovic, R., Kosanic, D., Ristic, B.: Noninvasive determination of knee cartilage deformation during jumping. J. Sports Sci. Med. **8**(4), 584 (2009)
3. Setuain, I., Martinikorena, J., Gonzalez-Izal, M., Martinez-Ramirez, A., Gómez, M., Alfaro-Adrián, J., Izquierdo, M.: Vertical jumping biomechanical evaluation through the use of an inertial sensor-based technology. J. Sports Sci. **34**, 1–9 (2015)
4. Mijailovic, N., Radakovic, R., Peulic, A., Milankovic, I., Filipovic, N.: Using force plate, computer simulation and image alignment in jumping analysis. In: 2015 IEEE 15th International Conference on Bioinformatics and Bioengineering (BIBE), Belgrade, pp. 1–4 (2015). https://doi.org/10.1109/bibe.2015.7367672
5. Hills, A., Hennig, E., McDonald, M., Bar-Or, O.: Plantar pressure differences between obese and non-obese adults: a biomechanical analysis. Int. J. Obes. **25**, 1674–1679 (2001)
6. Young, W.B., Behm, D.G.: Effects of running, static stretching and practice jumps on explosive force production and jumping performance. J. Sports Med. Phys. Fitness **43**(1), 21–27 (2003)
7. Omkar, S.N., Vanjare, A.M., Suhith, H., Kumar, G.H.: Motion analysis for short and long jump. Int. J. Perform. Anal. Sport **12**(1), 132–143 (2012)

# Numerical Modeling of Drug Delivery in Organs: From CT Scans to FE Model

Miljan Milosevic[1(✉)], Vladimir Simic[1], and Milos Kojic[1,2,3]

[1] Bioengineering Research and Development Center, BioIRC Kragujevac,
Prvoslava Stojanovica 6, 3400 Kragujevac, Serbia
miljan.m@kg.ac.rs, vladimir.simic.991@gmail.com,
mkojic42@gmail.com
[2] The Department of Nanomedicine, The Houston Methodist Research
Institute (TMHRI), 6670 Bertner Ave, Houston, TX 77030, USA
[3] Serbian Academy of Sciences and Arts,
Knez Mihailova 35, 11000 Belgrade, Serbia

**Abstract.** Mass transport within an organ is complex process which occurs through two different domains: networks of blood vessels and surrounding tissue. Consequently, development of a comprehensive transport model remains a challenge. In this paper we showed an application of a recently introduced multi-scale transport model [1, 2], where larger vessels are modeled by simple 1D finite elements. This model couples convective and diffusive transport within complex system consisted of capillaries and tissue, where connection between these fluid (capillaries) and solid (tissue) domains is accomplished by using fictitious 1D elements. In order to apply the developed model, a reconstruction procedure, consisted of: segmentation, skeletonization using augmented FMM method, and diameter recognition within indoor software, is processed. At the end, numerical simulations are performed in order to get the pressure and concentration distribution in the vessel network and surrounding tissue, showed by examples presented in the paper.

**Keywords:** Segmentation · Skeletonization · Finite element method
Pipe finite element · Pancreas model · Liver model

## 1 Introduction

Patient specific numerical modeling of drug transport in tumor and organs requires a long way from CT images to representative FE model. Models of tumor and organs are very complex due to heterogeneity of capillary network, tissue cells, etc. In order to have an accurate drug transport model, one would suggest that representation of complex capillary network should be done using either detailed 2D or 3D finite elements. But, it would be very demanding since the number of equations will increase rapidly, and process will soon become very inefficient.

We recently introduced a transport model which can be applied to large vascular systems [1, 2]. This model uses 1D finite element for larger vessels and equivalent continuum FEs for capillary beds. Additionally, the model incorporates blood vessel wall properties with respect to hydraulic and diffusive transport.

© ICST Institute for Computer Sciences, Social Informatics and Telecommunications Engineering 2018
N. Oliver et al. (Eds.): MindCare 2016/Fabulous 2016/IIoT 2015, LNICST 207, pp. 87–92, 2018.
https://doi.org/10.1007/978-3-319-74935-8_12

In our drug transport model [2], we considered that transport occurs from the arteries into tissue, and back - from tissue to the veins. First transport region is fluid domain consisting of blood, which is coupled with second region: solid (tissue) domain. We assume that transport of molecules, for both capillary and tissue domains, occurs by both convection and diffusion, by assumption that tissue is treated as a porous solid.

The most important part of generating realistic and accurate models for simulation of drug transport is to have appropriate tools. In order to create realistic model, a number of sub-steps have to be taken - from CT images to FE model. Our first step was the 3D segmentation from CT images using indoor CAD software. Next step was skeletonization of capillary objects, so capillaries can be used as 1D elements in the simulation. Skeletonization procedure is done using Augmented Fast Marching Method (FMM) [3, 4]. The reconstructed 1D trees of capillaries and the volumetric 3D model are then employed in numerical simulations of drug transport using the finite element method.

In Sect. 2 we summarize all methodologies implemented in our reconstruction process and modeling. In Sect. 3 we briefly formulate our computational model. At the end, in Sect. 4, we present results for two different examples: mouse pancreas and human liver models.

## 2    Reconstruction of the 3D Tissue and Capillary Network

The task of organ modeling, with detailed vasculature, can be divided in few sub-problems. First of all, geometry of larger vascular structures has to be identified from data obtained by CT scans.

Images are taken from CT scans, and reconstruction process is done using our CAD-Dicom software for 3D reconstruction. CAD-Dicom software is used for semi-automatic segmentation and generation of 3D meshes from dicom files (Fig. 1a). Graphical user interface of CAD-Dicom is build up using Visual Studio MFC classes. Meshes are then voxelised through a binvox application [3].

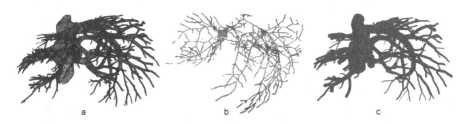

**Fig. 1.** (a) Segmentation process of liver model – 3D reconstruction of capillaries from CT images - mesh of outer faces; (b) Skeletonization of voxelized capillary network using SkeletonSandbox interface software [3]. (c) Diameter recognition of skeletonized lines using indoor CAD-Darcy graphical interface, according to voxelized capillary network.

In order to abstract from the voxel shape, various shape descriptors have been proposed. In 1967, Blum introduced the skeleton, which transforms a shape into another one that is of a lower dimensionality than the shape it describes [3]. Skeletons and medial axes can be produced in the three main ways: Morphological thinning, Geometric methods, and Distance transform (DT). A third class of methods computes the distance transform (DT) of the object's boundary. Recent approaches for computing the DT use the robust and simple implementation of Fast Marching Method (FMM) for evolution of boundaries in normal direction with constant speed.

In our model we used Skeleton sandbox software [3], and also algorithms based on Fast Marching Methods [4]. Skeleton Sandbox software uses a simple and robust method for computing skeletons for arbitrary planar objects and centerlines for 3D objects - Augmented FMM. Another algorithm based on FMM is available as open source Matlab code [4]. The resulting parameter field was then thresholded to produce the skeleton branches created by boundary features of a given size (Fig. 1b).

At the end, using our CAD-Darcy interface software, and algorithms for diameter recognition, we calculate diameters for each of pipe segments (Fig. 1c).

## 3  Fundamental FE Equations

In our recently introduced multi-scale transport model [1, 2] larger vessels are modeled by simple 1D finite elements, while capillary bed is modeled by equivalent 3D continuum finite elements. Introduced model couples convective–diffusive transport within fluid (capillaries) and solid (tissue) domain, where coupling is done using fictitious 1D finite element. Blood flow at lower hierarchies within tissue is modeled as parallel flows in a 3D porous media governed by the Darcy equation.

Blood vessel can be described as deformable pipe through which blood flows. In our paper [1] we formulated a 2-node finite element with deformable cross-section. In general, nodal variables can be pressures and nodal fluxes. From the continuity equation and the equation of the balance of linear momentum, the Navier-Stokes equation can be transformed into incremental-iterative FE balance equation, which can further be expressed for a time step $\Delta t$ and iteration $i$, as [5]:

$$\left(\mathbf{M}^{p(i-1)} + \mathbf{K}^{p(i-1)}\right)\Delta\mathbf{P}^{(i)} = \mathbf{F}^{(i-1)} - \left(\mathbf{M}^{p(i-1)} + \mathbf{K}^{p(i-1)}\right)\mathbf{P}^{(i-1)} + \mathbf{M}^{p(i-1)}\mathbf{P}^{t} \quad (1)$$

where the matrix components $M_{IJ}^{p(i-1)}$, $K_{IJ}^{p(i-1)}$ and $F_I^{(i-1)}$ are given in [2] in details, and $\mathbf{P}^{t}$ is nodal pressure at start of time step.

If we assume that blood can be considered as homogenous fluid, convective-diffusive transport within blood vessels will have mathematically very simplified form. In case of diffusion transport, in addition to (1) we will have another system of equations following from the balance equation of diffusion [2]:

$$\left(\frac{1}{\Delta t}\mathbf{M}^c + \mathbf{K}^c + \mathbf{K}^{cv}\right)^{(i-1)}\Delta\mathbf{C}^{(i)} = \mathbf{Q}_c^{ext} + \mathbf{Q}_c^V - \frac{1}{\Delta t}\mathbf{M}^{c(i-1)}\left(\mathbf{C}^{(i-1)} - \mathbf{C}^t\right)$$
$$- (\mathbf{K}^c + \mathbf{K}^{cv})^{(i-1)}\mathbf{C}^{(i-1)} \quad (2)$$

where the matrices $M_{IJ}^c$, $K_{IJ}^c$, $K_{IJ}^{cv}$ and the source vector $\mathbf{Q}_c^V$ are given in [2], and $\mathbf{C}^{(i-1)}$ and $\mathbf{C}^t$ are nodal concentrations at the iteration $(i - 1)$ and start of time step, respectively; $\mathbf{Q}_c^{ext}$ is the external nodal flux vector, and $\mathbf{K}^{cv}$ is matrix which couples convection and diffusion within the pipe.

The boundary between fluid and tissue domain is represented by blood vessel walls. As was extensively investigated in the past, particulate transport through the wall is very complex due to various physical and biological effects. In order to overcome those challenges, we in [2] introduced 2-node 1D fictitious elements which can connect these two domains. For each of those domains, in practical applications, we select continuum nodes which are connected to the 1D pipe elements. Introduced 1D fictitious element includes all wall transport properties, regarding diffusion and convection transport. Additional details regarding the implementation of fictitious 1D elements and connection between domains are given in [2].

## 4   Results

In following two examples we present applications of our numerical model for large systems consisted of blood vessels and tissue: one for a mouse pancreas and the other for a human liver. Data were obtained by CT imaging at Huston Methodist Research Institute, and at MD Anderson Cancer Center, Houston, USA. The computational models were generated at the R&D Center for Bioengineering, Kragujevac, Serbia and implemented into our FE code PAK [6].

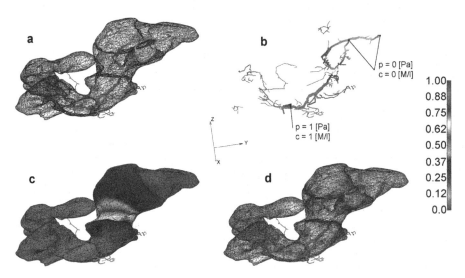

**Fig. 2.** Numerical model of pancreas vasculature and tissue. Pressure field for first (t = 2.5 s) time step of simulation. (a) 1D vascular network together with 3D mesh, (b) 1D mesh with prescribed values for pressures, (c) Full 3D mesh of tissue, (d) 1D vascular network together with 3D mesh – 3D results represented by dots.

Both models are composed of 1D finite elements representing blood vessels, fictitious elements to connect fluid and tissue domain, and 3D elements for tissue. Prescribed values for blood vessels are inlet/outlet pressures and inlet/outlet concentrations (Figs. 2b and 3c). Input parameters for both models are: Inlet pressure is 1 Pa, Outlet pressure is 0 Pa, Inlet concentration is 1 M/L, Outlet concentration is 0, Viscosity of fluid is $10^{-3}$ Pa s, Leakage coefficient of vessel wall is $10^{-11}$ mm/s (convection through vessel wall), Diffusion coefficient in vessels is $10^4$ mm$^2$/s, Diffusion coefficient in 3D tissue is 0.5 mm$^2$/s, and Darcy coefficient in 3D tissue is $10^{-15}$ mm$^2$/Pa s.

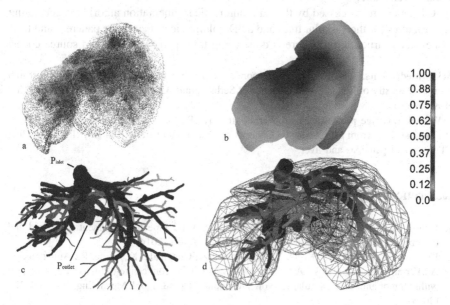

**Fig. 3.** Numerical model of human liver: (a) Pressure field for first (t = 2.5 s) time step of simulation - 1D vascular network together with 3D mesh (3D results represented by dots), (b) Concentration field for t = 2.5 s - full 3D mesh of tissue, (c) 1D mesh with prescribed values for pressures, (d) Concentration distribution - 1D vascular network with outer mesh of 3D model.

The pressure distribution within tissue and capillary network is shown in Fig. 2 for mouse pancreas model, and Fig. 3a and c for human liver, where the pressure changes from the inlet artery to the outlet vein. The concentration field is displayed in Figs. 3b and d, where concentration gradients are evident from the region of inlet artery to the region of outlet vein. The presented results for pressure and concentration fields show applicability of the presented model to other specific organs.

## 5   Conclusion

The goal of this study was to describe challenges in 3D reconstruction of complex geometries, such as tumors or human organs, and also in generating accurate computational model which is feasible for simulation of mass transport within those domains, consisted of large blood vessel networks. We used recently formulated and computationally efficient 1D pipe finite element for blood vessels [1], which can take into account wall deformability in a simplified form. To couple transport between blood vessels and surrounding tissues we used recently introduced fictitious 1D finite element [2], which accounts for the hydraulic and diffusive properties of the vessel walls.

Presented computational methodology was implemented into our FE code PAK [6] - a research code developed over decades. The listed numerical concepts, which form the basis of our model, are implemented in two different examples: mouse pancreas and human liver model.

CT data were processed by the semi-automatic segmentation algorithms generating 1D structures for the vascular trees and a 3D volumetric model of the pancreas and liver tissue. Reconstruction procedure is done using third party software and source codes.

**Acknowledgments.** This work was supported in part by the Houston Methodist Research Institute, Ministry of Education and Science of Serbia, grants OI 174028 and III 41007, and City of Kragujevac.

We acknowledge professor Mauro Ferrari from HMRI for overall leadership and guidance, Dr. Eugene Koay from MD Anderson Cancer Center and Sara Errani from HMRI for providing CT images of pancreas and liver.

# References

1. Kojic, M., Milosevic, M., Simic, V., Ferrari, M.: A 1D pipe finite element with rigid and deformable walls. J. Serb. Soc. Comput. Mech. **8**, 38–53 (2014)
2. Kojic, M., Milosevic, M., Kojic, N., Starosolski, Z., Ghaghada, K., Serda, R., Annapragada, A., Ferrari, M., Ziemys, A.: A multi-scale FE model for convective-diffusive drug transport within tumor and large vascular networks. Comput. Methods Appl. Mech. Eng. **294**, 100–122 (2015)
3. Reniers, D., van Wijk, J.J., Telea, A.: Computing multiscale curve and surface skeletons of genus 0 shapes using a global importance measure. IEEE Trans. Visual. Comput. Graph. **14** (2), 355–368 (2008)
4. van Uitert, R., Bitter, I.: Subvoxel precise skeletons of volumetric data base on fast marching methods (2007)
5. Kojic, M., Filipovic, N., Stojanovic, B., Kojic, N.: Computer Modeling in Bioengineering - Theoretical Background, Examples and Software. Wiley, Chichester (2008)
6. Kojic, M., Slavkovic, R., Zivkovic, M., Grujovic, N., Filipovic, N.: PAK—Finite Element Program for Linear and Nonlinear Analysis. University of Kragujevac, R&D Center for Bioengineering Kragujevac, Serbia (1998, 2010)

# FPGA Implementation of Face Recognition Algorithm

Tijana Šušteršič[✉], Aleksandra Vulović, Nenad Filipović,
and Aleksandar Peulić

Faculty of Engineering, University of Kragujevac,
Sestre Janjić 6, 34 000 Kragujevac, Serbia
{tijanas, aleksandra.vulovic, fica,
aleksandar.peulic}@kg.ac.rs

**Abstract.** Field of face recognition has been developing in the past several decades. Although percentage of successful recognition algorithms is constantly getting higher, there is room for improvement. Field Programmable Gate Array (FPGA) is technology that can be used for speed and accuracy improvement. The main goal of this paper was to load photos from files to FPGA and display, as well as describe implementation of the Eigenface algorithm on DE2 Altera board. We showed that DE2 Altera board can be used for reading databases and photos from crime scenes and discussed how Eigenface algorithm can be implemented on this board in order to speed up the process of face recognition. Speed of recognition process is an area where improvement is necessary, especially considering the need for instant face recognition in places like airports, or public meetings.

**Keywords:** FPGA · Face recognition · Eigenface algorithm

## 1 Introduction

In recent years, researches in face recognition techniques have gained significant momentum [1]. Though it is much easier to install face recognition system in a large setting, the actual implementation is very challenging as it needs to account for all possible appearance variation caused by change in illumination, facial features, variations in pose, image resolution, sensor noise, viewing distance, occlusions, etc. [2].

In the past decade, an increased number of requests was addressed to forensic expert witnesses in Serbia with the focus on verification of the identity of individuals presented on video or images available from crime scenes. Mainly due to budgetary constraints, Serbia did not develop any automatic or semiautomatic system for face recognition. Practically, when the police and court obtain image-based evidence from video surveillance cameras, forensic experts are only left with manual analyses. Moreover, the process is limited to few experienced forensic experts and their traditional anthropological approach which is not based on objective measurements. The method lacks consistent methodology and there is a great need to standardize the process. Moreover, the numerous studies show that using human perception alone (e.g. eye witnessing) is not always a reliable source to confirm identification, and is

© ICST Institute for Computer Sciences, Social Informatics and Telecommunications Engineering 2018
N. Oliver et al. (Eds.): MindCare 2016/Fabulous 2016/IIoT 2015, LNICST 207, pp. 93–99, 2018.
https://doi.org/10.1007/978-3-319-74935-8_13

significantly affected by differences in lighting, familiarity, expression and viewpoint or pose [3]. The application of face recognition techniques can be categorized into two main parts: law enforcement application and commercial application. Law enforcement applications would include identification of wanted individuals, while the commercial applications range from static matching of photographs on credit cards, ATM cards, passports, driver's licenses, and photo ID to real-time matching with still images or video image sequences for access control. Each application presents different constraints in terms of processing [4]. Most viable application in the area of law enforcement is at the airports and in transportation (e.g. airports, train stations, border crossings). There is also an application in public security systems (e.g. criminal identification, digital driver license) [5]. Commercial use of face recognition can be found in identification systems (e.g. automatic banking, computer log-in, etc.) [5] and gaming (e.g. keeping out the compulsive gamblers).

Among different types of algorithms for face recognition, those that are simple, and at the same time efficient, stand out. In high-dimensional data, the Principal Component Analysis (PCA) is designed to model linear variation. Its goal is to find a set of mutually orthogonal basis functions that capture the directions of maximum variance in the data and for which the coefficients are pairwise decorrelated [6]. PCA was used to describe face images in terms of a set of basic functions, or "eigenfaces". Eigenfaces was introduced early on [7] as a powerful use of PCA to solve problems in face recognition and detection. Principal component analysis for face recognition is based on the information theory approach in which the relevant information in a face image is extracted as efficiently as possible [8].

Most of the available algorithms are implemented in software. As a result, the recognition speed is not as expected [9]. On the other hand, hardware implementation such as Field Programmable Gate Array (FPGA) has many promises. In recent years, people have made effort to apply it to biology and neuroscience due to its favorable performance [9]. Compared with the software simulation, FPGA shows more advantages over PC-solution. First, parallel processing of FPGA significantly improves computational efficiency, which effectively solves the time-consuming problem in a general-purpose system. Second, because of its re-configurable nature, FPGA implementation allows for development of a module repertoire which includes a variety of neuron models for different purposes [10].

The DE2 board has many features that allow a user to implement a wide range of designed circuits, from simple circuits to various multimedia projects. DE2 board used in this paper has Altera Cyclone® II 2C35 FPGA device (Fig. 1).

It has Altera Serial Configuration device – EPCS16, USB Blaster, 512-KB SRAM, 8-MB SDRAM, 4-MB Flash memory, SD Card socket, 4 pushbutton switches, 18 toggle switches, 9 green user LEDs, 50-MHz oscillator and 27-MHz oscillator for clock sources, VGA DAC with VGA out connector, RS-232 transceiver, PS/2 mouse/keyboard connector, two 40-pin Expansion Headers with diode protection [11].

Therefore, our motivation was to load face photos from AT&T database and to discuss hardware implementation of the Eigenface algorithm in a Cyclone II Field Programmable Gate Array (FPGA) chip from Altera Inc.

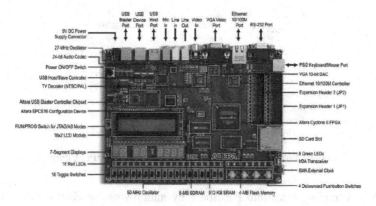

**Fig. 1.** The DE2 board

## 2 Materials and Methods

Material used for this paper was AT&T database which consisted of grayscale photos of 40 people, where each person was photographed 10 times (400 photos on the whole). These 10 photos of each person were made at different times, varying the lighting, facial expressions (open/closed eyes, smiling/not smiling) and facial details (glasses/no glasses). All the images were taken against a dark homogeneous background with the subjects in an upright, frontal position (with tolerance for some side movement). Each image had the size of $112 \times 92$ pixels with 256 levels of grey.

FPGA can be used to implement any logical function that an application-specific integrated circuit (ASIC) could perform. Unlike previous generation FPGAs using I/Os with programmable logic and interconnects, today's FPGAs consist of various mixes of configurable embedded SRAM, high-speed transceivers, high-speed I/Os, logic blocks, and routing. We used that property of writing from a file to SRAM to load any photo from AT&T database into the FPGA's SRAM memory and display it on a computer monitor connected to an FPGA via VGA video port.

In order to implement an Eigenface algorithm, we have to load the database and the photo from crime scene. This is done by storing the photos in chip memory and processing the images with Eigenface algorithm using Nios II after which the results are displayed on a computer monitor (Fig. 2).

Furthermore, we present Eigenface algorithm for face recognition image processing implemented on a FPGA.

*Implementation of the Eigenface algorithm*

*Step 1.* Identification by eigen faces

a. Compute the average face
b. Subtract the average face from the training faces
c. Compute covariance matrix
d. Determine eigenvectors and eigenvalues
e. Choose a certain number of eigenvectors with highest eigenvalues

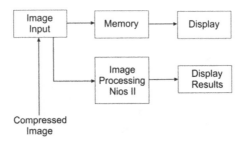

**Fig. 2.** Block diagram of image processing on a FPGA chip

f. Project training faces into Facespace by multiplying the eigenvectors with the matrix obtained in the step 1-b.

*Step 2.* Recognition by matching eigen faces

a. Subtract the average face from the face
b. Compute the projection into Facespace by multiplying the eigenvectors with the matrix obtained in the step 2-a
c. Compute the threshold based on the distance in the face space between the face and all known faces by using Euclidian distance.

*Step 3.* Categorization of the result by grouping

a. Distinguish between the cases based on the threshold obtained in step 2-c
   I. It is an unknown face (person is not in database) - update the database with this face and inform the user that it is an unknown face
   II. It is a known face (person is already in database) - inform the user what are the possibilities and probabilities for correct recognition (pick three photo matches with shortest Euclidian distance).

It can be seen that the operations in Eigenface algorithm include simple mathematical operations with huge matrices. In cases of even greater databases, the speed of recognition is relatively small. An FPGA can provide us with necessary resources to achieve such improvements in face recognition process speedup. The resources include built in blocks, various communication interfaces, millions of logic gates, scopes to run C codes into the digital hardware circuitry, high level design tools, performance, long term maintenance, reliability, etc. The cyclone chip is relatively cheaper and includes ROM. DE0 board has been chosen as a tool for debugging process. We have only discussed implementation of Eigenface algorithm.

## 3 Results and Discussion

One of the prime concerns of our research was to start with the simpler algorithm, to confirm that it was possible to implement other, more complicated, algorithms using FPGA, so that we can work on it in future.

To achieve implementation of Eigenface algorithm on Altera Cyclotrone II FPGA, a processor using Qsys needs to be created. Various components such as CPU, SDRAM, PLL, Tri state bridge, Onchip memory, etc. need to be added. Connection by connecting master to slave, source to sink, assigned base address and connected clock through PLL needs to be made.

The result of writing a file to an SRAM displaying it on a computer monitor connected to an FPGA via VGA video port is given in Fig. 3. The visualization was achieved using Quartus II 13.0 which was used in order to run the DE2 Control Panel throughout which the image was loaded and stored in SRAM memory as well as for the SRAM controller the User Port 1 (Asynchronous 1) is chosen.

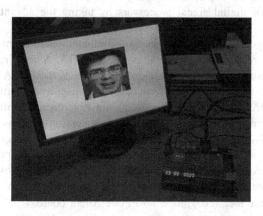

**Fig. 3.** Displaying loaded photo on a computer monitor connected to an FPGA

Next step would be to write Verilog/VHDL code to interface in our FPGA through pin assignment. Then we should include our SOPC code in Verilog/VHDL code and interface with our board's pin which generates the .SOF file. That would complete the hardware configuration. Another possibility is to write our Matlab code for Eigenface algorithm and convert it to HDL code. We showed that it was possible to load any photo to an FPGA which can be further used in the process of recognition.

The time constraints of our system are bounded by the time constraints required by real time face recognition. That is, in applications where the recognition of multiple faces is required, the process must not take more than 2 s for each person. However, this process includes the overhead of obtaining the image, performing face recognition, and displaying the results. Normally, using CPU, the face recognition process is in the order of milliseconds when working with small databases. Logical parallelism within an image processing operation is well suited to FPGA implementation when working with large databases, and it is here where many image processing algorithms may be accelerated significantly. This is accomplished by unrolling the inner loops, so that rather than performing the operations sequentially, parallel hardware is used.

Prior to obtaining any measurements, we developed a hypothesis that the projection phase would consume the longest portion of time. This assumption stemmed from the fact that this phase involves high computational demand in the form of a matrix multiplication operation. In [9] it took approximately 10% less clock cycles to execute face recognition algorithm using hardware FPGA than the software implementation.

## 4 Conclusion

FPGA is a piece of hardware that implements thousands of gates of logic that are preferably used when the speed up in the design process is desired. Using hardware programming languages such as VHDL and Verilog someone can create complex logic structures. Speed is the biggest advantage of FPGA. It is reprogrammable so that more than one project can be implemented using same FPGA board. FPGAs exceed the computing power of digital signal processors by taking the advantage of hardware parallelism.

Therefore, our goal was to outline the possibilities of implementation of a simple algorithm for face recognition – Eigenface on a FPGA. Since the algorithm itself includes simple mathematical operations, total benefits of the FPGA can be obtained. We loaded photos from the AT&T database and displayed them on a computer monitor. Furthermore, we gave the pseudo code for Eigenface algorithm which will be used in order to perform face recognition image processing by Nios II.

However, FPGAs are more expensive than microcontrollers. If the designed problem needs greater integration density, then FPGAs are appropriate. For smaller projects, microcontrollers would be a better solution. For the purpose of creating the Face recognition system in Serbia, FPGAs would greatly help. Future work with FPGA will include real time face recognition on FPGA Altera board.

## References

1. Li, Z.S.: Encyclopedia of Biometrics. Springer, New York (2009)
2. Surti, R.N., Rodrigues, A.: Performance evaluation of statistical approaches of face recognition techniques. Int. J. Statistika Mathematika 10, 08–11 (2014)
3. Smeets, D., Claes, P., Vandermeulen, D., Clement, J.G.: Objective 3D face recognition: evolution, approaches and challenges. Forensic Sci. Int. 201, 125–132 (2010)
4. Tolba, A.S., El-Baz, A.H., El-Harby, A.A.: Face recognition: a literature review. Int. J. Sig. Process. 2, 88–103 (2006)
5. Mou, D.: Machine-Based Intelligent Face Recognition. Springer, Heidelberg (2010)
6. Ragab, A., Albert, C., Senousy, M.B.: A comparative study of face recognition techniques. Int. J. Electron. Commun. Comput. Eng. 6, 762–770 (2015)
7. Turk, M., Pentland, A.: Eigenfaces for recognition. J. Cogn. Neurosci. 3, 71–86 (1991)
8. Agarwal, M., Agrawal, H., Jain, N., Kumar, M.: Face recognition using principle component analysis, eigenface and neural network. In: International Conference on Signal Acquisition and Processing (ICSAP 2010), pp. 310–314. IEEE Computer Society (2010)
9. Dewan, P.D., Shamma, T.H., Abbas, A., Mondol, R.K.: Design and VLSI implementation of high performance face recognition system. A report submitted to department of Electrical & Electronic Engineering, BRAC University in partial fulfillment of the requirements for thesis work (2013)

10. Eric Deng, V.P.: Accelerator for POWER, revolutionizing the datacenter. In: Open Power Summit, San Jose, CA, 5–8 April 2016
11. Terasic Technologies: Development and Education Board DE2, User Manual (2006). https://www.terasic.com.tw

# Persons Counting and Monitoring System Based on Passive Infrared Sensors and Ultrasonic Sensors (PIRUS)

Ana-Maria Claudia Drăgulinescu, Ioana Marcu, Simona Halunga,
and Octavian Fratu$^{(\boxtimes)}$ ⓘ

Telecommunications Department, Electronics, Telecommunications
and Information Technology Faculty, University "Politehnica" of Bucharest,
Bucharest, Romania
amc.dragulinescu@gmail.com, ofratu@elcom.pub.ro

**Abstract.** Counting systems are widely used for applications related to counting people within a certain area or traffic monitoring in a crowded commercial area, for automatic settings of air-conditioning systems depending on the number of the persons located in that space, etc. Persons counting and identification systems are useful in educational domain or in cultural and entertaining areas where resource allocation must treat differently every class of customers. Therefore the main goal of the paper is to present a sensor-based system that can be used either to monitor the presence of the students in a classroom or to differentially count adults and children that enter parks, museums, etc. The implemented system (PIRUS) comprises passive infrared sensors and ultrasonic sensors. Multiple scenarios have been depicted in order to analyze and improve the performances of the designed system.

**Keywords:** Persons counting · PIR · Ultrasonic · Height discrimination

## 1 Introduction

People counting and classifying systems are necessary tools in many daily situations, such as registering the students' attendance to courses, estimating the presence of people that belong to different age categories (adults-children) in order to provide different services or to improve the quality of the existing ones according to the customer profile. Counting systems may comprise modules of sensors of the same type [1, 2] or several types of sensors in the so-called fusion-based sensor based networks [3–5]. These systems may also use vision-based motion sensors [6] or motion sensors based on other technologies, such as passive infrared sensors and pressure mats [3]. As opposed to vision sensors, passive infrared sensors are mass- produced at low costs [7] and are non-intrusive. For relevant results, though, PIR sensors must be used together with other types of technologies, sensors and/or devices. However, there is a need for continuous research as the real world scenarios modify and new issues must be solved.

This paper proposes to configure a low-cost counting and discriminating system based on a minimum number of passive infrared and ultrasonic sensors. The paper is

© ICST Institute for Computer Sciences, Social Informatics and Telecommunications Engineering 2018
N. Oliver et al. (Eds.): MindCare 2016/Fabulous 2016/IIoT 2015, LNICST 207, pp. 100–106, 2018.
https://doi.org/10.1007/978-3-319-74935-8_14

organized as follows: Sect. 2 briefly describes the functioning principle of the motion sensors used. In Sect. 3, we mention the parameters that may be extracted using the two types of sensors and we present the people counting and discrimination system diagram, explaining its functioning. We also include the experiments and the results of four different scenarios through which we tested the system. Section 4 presents our conclusions and future research prospects.

## 2 Motion Sensors Used for Human Tracking, Counting and Discrimination

### 2.1 Passive Infrared Sensors (PIR)

Passive Infrared Sensors are sensitive to infrared radiation modification, that is, to the heat exchange between the sensing elements and moving body [8]. They are designed to consider only radiation in a certain domain, specific to human body thermal radiation (7–14 μm). In this paper, we considered Passive Infrared Sensor from Pololu [9]. The functioning principle presented for this sensor is valid also for other PIRs. The sensor has a dual sensing element based on both metal and pyroelectric films whose polarization changes as the temperature changes due to pyroelectric phenomenon. In response to the material heating, a temporary voltage will be generated on each sensing element [10]. When a (human) being passes in front of the sensor orthogonal on the sensing elements, they are sequentially activated and the motion is detected.

### 2.2 Ultrasonic Sensors (US)

Ultrasonic sensors are distance measuring sensors based on reverse piezoelectric effect [8]. They produce ultrasonic bursts that may be sent to a target through their emitters. When arriving on the target, the wave reflects and goes back to its receiver. The received wave is converted in a voltage. The parameter of interest is the travelling time. Knowing the speed of sound, duration may be translated into distance. There are different output interfaces for an ultrasonic sensor (TTL, RS232, Analogue and PWM [11, 12]). In this paper we chose LV EZ4 Sensor from MaxBotix [12] and PWM output interface. This means that the travelling time is given by the duration of logic "1". The distance is computed using the scale factor given by manufacturers.

## 3 PIRUS System Parameters, Diagram and Testing

Motion speed, distance with respect to sensor and persons dimensions may significantly influence PIR sensors output [1]. In this paper, we analyse the PIR output in order to extract information about direction of target.

The output of US gives information about the presence and even on the dimensions of the target in its field of view. This happens due to its narrow beam width which allows the detection of persons up to approximately 121.92 cm (4 ft).

Figure 1 presents the disposal of the two sensors at an entrance of 70 × 200 cm. US is placed at the middle of the upper door case, considering that US board has 1.99 × 2.21 cm. PIR sensor is placed on the left lateral part of door case, at a height of 70 cm.

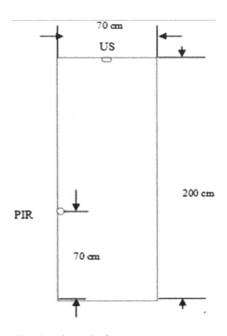

**Fig. 1.** Disposal of sensors at an entrance

The flowchart of the proposed system is depicted in Fig. 2. The system is based on Arduino Uno Prototyping Platform and IDE. For monitoring the sensors' output signals, we used both Serial Monitoring provided by Arduino IDE and Arduino Support Package for MATLAB. In the initialisation step, PIR and US are calibrated. The latter sends an initial burst for achieving the distance between the sensor output (found at 1.55 cm below the door case or at 198.45 cm above the ground) and bottom part of the door case found at 0 cm because it was embedded in the floor. After initialisation, the two low-power sensors are interrogated continuously. In a first experiment, three sets of 20 initialisation readings were done in order to verify the accuracy of the readings. For every set, we computed the average and the relative error of the average with respect to the real value, 198.45 cm (Table 1).

The results in Table 1 reveal inaccuracy of US and non-constant relative error, which is very important for discrimination issue. This happens due to the fact that US output depends on medium changes (temperature and humidity) and the scale factor for distance computation considers the standard sound speed of 345.57 m/s instead of following the environmental changes. In a future work, this aspect will be improved.

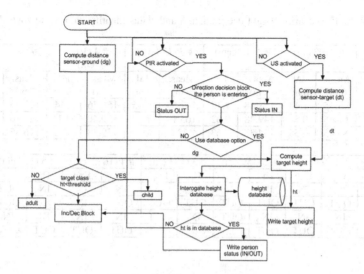

**Fig. 2.** PIRUS system diagram

**Table 1.** Measurement sets for initialisation step

| Measurement set | Average [cm] | Relative error [%] |
|---|---|---|
| I | 198.40 | 0.025 |
| II | 200.00 | 0.781 |
| III | 200.15 | 0.856 |

The previous experiments showed that US is not able to detect targets with small surfaces (e.g. children with height less than 85 cm, because of their small shoulders width and not because of their height!). One may consider this as a disadvantage, but we fructified this using the information given by PIR. Thus, if US is not triggered (ht = 0 < threshold), but only PIR, we considered a child entered.

PIR output signal is analyzed and a function is implemented in order to fulfil the *direction decision block*. At this stage of research, we do not take into account the occlusion phenomenon, i.e., when many persons pass simultaneously. According to the diagram, the system offers two extra options: either counting and identifying persons already registered in a database or counting differentially adults and children.

In order to test the system, we realized four scenarios and each of them was reproduced in order to obtain at least 3 sets of experimental results for each scenario.

*In the first scenario*, 5 persons (2 children and 3 adults) entered one after the other. We gathered information about their heights (if available) and direction. The results are tabulated in Table 2. The heights absolute error was computed as the difference between theoretical and experimental values. We observed that lower absolute values were obtained for smaller subjects. We showed, thus, that at this moment, the system must consider deviations x = 9.62 cm in order to work properly. This means that it is not suitable to discriminate between persons whose heights differ with less than

**Table 2.** 1$^{st}$ scenario. Height determination and status identification (inside/outside)

| Set | | # 1 (93 cm) | | # 2 (159 cm) | | # 3 (173 cm) | | # 4 (162.5 cm) | | # 5 (127 cm) | |
|---|---|---|---|---|---|---|---|---|---|---|---|
| Cm | % | Meas. (cm) | \|Δ\| (cm) | Meas. (cm) | \|Δ\| (cm) | Meas. (cm) | \|Δ\| (cm) | Meas. (cm) | \|Δ\| (cm) | Meas. (cm) | \|Δ\| (cm) |
| I | | 94.45 | 1.45 | 151.88 | 7.12 | 167.54 | 5.46 | 156.76 | 5.74 | 121.96 | 5.04 |
| II | | 92.45 | 0.55 | 149.38 | 9.62 | 165.19 | 7.81 | 159.40 | 3.1 | 124.36 | 2.64 |
| III | | 89.45 | 3.55 | 154.37 | 4.63 | 172.6 | 0.4 | 159.38 | 3.12 | 126.85 | 0.15 |

| Set | | # 1 (93 cm) | | # 2 (159 cm) | | # 3 (173 cm) | | # 4 (162.5 cm) | | # 5 (127 cm) | |
|---|---|---|---|---|---|---|---|---|---|---|---|
| | | Th. | Exp | Th. | Exp | Th. | Exp | Th. | Exp | Th. | Exp |
| I | | IN | IN | IN | IN | IN | OUT | IN | IN | IN | OUT |
| II | | OUT | OUT | OUT | OUT | OUT | OUT | OUT | IN | OUT | OUT |
| III | | IN | IN | IN | OUT | IN | OUT | IN | IN | IN | IN |
| IV | | OUT | OUT | OUT | OUT | OUT | OUT | OUT | OUT | OUT | OUT |

9.62 cm, as in the cases #2 and #4. Using such a threshold, #2 was always confounded with 4. Also, we applied median filtering of absolute errors and we assigned a value m = 3.55 cm for the deviation. In only 33.3% of cases #2 was correctly identified. #4 was always confounded with #2 for this value. This is why we chose finally a value of x − m = 6.58 cm for which #2 and #4 are recognized correctly. In what concerns the direction of movement, the system recognized correctly 15/20 events.

*In the second scenario*, using the data in Table 2 (real heights and absolute errors) we stored the heights in a database with appropriate height deflection and the task of the system was to recognize the persons that entered by their heights.

Table 3 comprises the results of *the third scenario*, in which the system had to classify the target as adult or child. The considered abbreviations in Table 3 are: I- person identified = YES/NO, #Passing order, T-Theoretical, E-Experimental determination, C-child, A-adult.

**Table 3.** 2$^{nd}$/3$^{rd}$ scenario. Person identification using database and discrimination adult/child

| Set | # 1 (93 cm) | | | | # 2 (159 cm) | | | | # 3 (173 cm) | | | | # 4 (162.5 cm) | | | | # 5 (127 cm) | | | |
|---|---|---|---|---|---|---|---|---|---|---|---|---|---|---|---|---|---|---|---|---|
| | # | I | T | E | # | I | T | E | # | I | T | E | # | I | T | E | # | I | T | E |
| I | 2 | Y | C | C | 3 | Y | A | A | 1 | Y | A | A | 5 | Y | A | A | 4 | Y | C | C |
| II | 5 | Y | C | C | 4 | Y | A | A | 3 | Y | A | A | 2 | Y | A | A | 1 | Y | C | C |
| III | 3 | Y | C | C | 5 | Y | A | A | 4 | Y | A | A | 1 | Y | A | A | 2 | Y | C | C |
| IV | 4 | Y | C | C | 1 | Y | A | A | 2 | Y | A | A | 3 | Y | A | A | 5 | Y | C | C |

*The last scenario* implies four or less persons, entering or exiting with a delay of 1 s one after the other. The system had to approach the event and to return the number of persons (Table 4).

**Table 4.** 4th scenario. People counting testing (Delay IN, Delay OUT = 1 s between passers-by

| Set | IN | OUT | Th. No. | | Exp. No. | | Percentage [%] |
|-----|------|-------|----|-----|----|-----|---------------|
| | | | IN | OUT | IN | OUT | |
| I | #1 | #3 | 1 | 1 | 1 | 1 | 100 |
| II | #2,#3 | #4 | 2 | 1 | 2 | 1 | 100 |
| III | #1,#2 | #3,#4 | 2 | 2 | 2 | 2 | 100 |
| IV | #2,#3,#1 | #4 | 1 | 3 | 1 | 1 | 50% |

## 4 Conclusions and Future Research

The paper emphasizes the work and results concerning the design of a people counting and discriminating system. By using PIR sensors and US, we developed a low-cost system aimed to provide information about the number of persons that enter or exit a place by extracting the motion direction parameter with a success rate of 75%. Moreover, the system may recognize passers-by through their height with a result of 100%, if information regarding their height is stored in a database and if we use the difference between maximum and median value of absolute errors in order to obtain the deviation. Also, the system may discriminate between adults and children with the same promising results of 100% if a threshold of 145 cm is chosen. We succeeded in counting persons that enter and exit in different numbers with a percentage of 100% when two or fewer people entered or exited with a small delay of 1 s and a success rate of 50% when more than two persons exited or entered with the same delay.

Future plans include enhancement of our system and its capabilities by considering the variation of the speed of sound with respect to medium conditions for the ultrasonic measurements. Also, we propose improving the extraction of the motion direction parameter using a more specialized method of comparing the output signal samples.

**Acknowledgments.** This work has been funded by European Commission by FP7 IP project no. 610658/2013 "eWALL for Active Long Living – eWALL" and by UEFISCDI Romania under Grant No. 20/2012 "Scalable Radio Transceiver for Instrumental Wireless Sensor Networks", SaRaT-IWSN and support grant no. 262EU/2013 "eWALL". The authors thank to Grayling Romania for their kind financial support in the present paper submission and presentation.

## References

1. Zappi, P., Farella, E., Benini, L.: Tracking motion direction and distance with pyroelectric IR sensors. IEEE Sens. J. **10**(9), 1486–1494 (2010)
2. Yun, J., Lee, S.S.: Human movement detection and identification using pyroelectric infrared sensors. Sens. J. **14**(5), 8057–8081 (2014)

3. Al-Naimi, I., Wong, C.B., Moore, P., Chen X.: Advanced approach for indoor identification and tracking using smart floor and pyroelectric infrared sensors. In: 5th International Conference on Information and Communication Systems (ICICS), Irbid, pp. 1–6 (2014)
4. Dan, B.-K., Kim, Y.-S., Suryanto, C.H., Jung, J.-Y., Ko, S.-J.: Robust people counting system based on sensor fusion. IEEE Trans. Consum. Electron. **58**(3), 1013–1021 (2012)
5. Luo, R.C., Chen, O., Lin C.W.: Indoor human monitoring system using wireless and pyroelectric sensory fusion system. In: 2010 IEEE/RSJ International Conference Intelligent Robots and Systems, Taipei, pp. 1507–1512 (2010)
6. Coşkun, A., Kara, A., Parlaktuna, M., Ozkan, M., Parlaktuna, O.: People counting system by using kinect sensor. In: 2015 International Symposium on Innovations in Intelligent SysTems and Applications, Madrid, pp. 1–7 (2015)
7. Wahl, F., Milenkovic, M., Amft, O.: A green autonomous self-sustaining sensor node for counting people in office environments. In: Proceedings of the 5th European DSP Education and Research Conference (EDERC), Amsterdam, pp. 203–207 (2012)
8. Fraden, J.: Handbook of Modern Sensors. Springer Science + Business Media, LLC, New York (2010)
9. Pololu Robotics and Electronics. https://www.pololu.com/product/1635
10. Sinclair, I.R.: Sensors and Transducers. Newnes Publishing House, Oxford (2001)
11. Parallax Inc. https://www.parallax.com/sites/default/files/downloads/28015-PING-Sensor-Product-Guide-v2.0.pdf
12. MaxBotix Inc. http://www.maxbotix.com/documents/MB1040_Datasheet.pdf

# Personalized and Intelligent Sleep Lifestyle Reasoner with Web Application for Improving Quality of Sleep Part of AAL Architecture

Krasimir Tonchev, Georgi Tsenov, Valeri Mladenov,
Agata Manolova(✉), and Vladimir Poulkov

Faculty of Telecommunications, Technical University of Sofia,
8 Kliment Ohridski blvd., 1000 Sofia, Bulgaria
{k_tonchev,gogotzenov,valerim,
amanolova,vkp}@tu-sofia.bg

**Abstract.** An average human spends about one third of his life sleeping so quality of sleep is essential for the human being to maintain good physical and emotional health. Sleep disorders may introduce severe physical effects, e.g. cognitive impairments and mental health complications. So being able to measure and evaluate sleep behavior is important for health practitioners and the users themselves. In this paper, we present the implementation of the Sleep Lifestyle Reasoner part of AAL platform which allows detection of minor or major deviations in the sleeping patterns in MCI and COPD patients indicating changes in their health status. The output of the reasoner is fed to the My Sleep Web Application that provides recommendations to improve sleep hygiene and coaches the users into a healthy sleeping behavior, based on their personal rhythms and problems. It also supports the informal caregiver by providing insights on the sleeping behavior of the patient.

**Keywords:** Intelligent Decision Support System · Sleep quality
Sleep monitoring · Context awareness · Ambient Assisted Living

## 1 Introduction

It is estimated that around twenty five per cent of elderly people worldwide have sleeping disorders [1]. Bad nights of sleep make people feel tired during the day, lose their enthusiasm and get easily irritated. Insufficient sleep is also associated with significant morbidity and increased mortality [2], and with an increased risk of falls [3]. Insomnia becomes a more common problem with age.

Along with the common sleep disorders related to the ageing population, detection of sleep disturbances in elderly suffering from Mild Cognitive Impairments (MCI) may be a predictive marker of the conditions' progression [4]. An irregular sleep–wake pattern can reflect the level of cognitive impairment. As the disease progresses, more severe sleep disturbances develop which affect the continuity of nighttime sleep, alertness during the day and overall wellbeing. The evaluation of sleep disturbances can help toward a proper diagnosis and a better understanding of the cognitive condition of the person with cognitive impairments [5].

© ICST Institute for Computer Sciences, Social Informatics and Telecommunications Engineering 2018
N. Oliver et al. (Eds.): MindCare 2016/Fabulous 2016/IIoT 2015, LNICST 207, pp. 107–112, 2018.
https://doi.org/10.1007/978-3-319-74935-8_15

The increasing inclusion of the new technologies in the everyday life of people more precisely the Ambient Assisted Living (AAL) architecture, provides an ecosystem of different types of sensors, computers, mobile devices, wireless networks and software applications for personal healthcare monitoring systems [6]. In recent years a number of smart home projects based on AAL have been developed [7]. In some of these home health-care systems automatic sleep monitoring platforms using different kinds of sensors and data processing are developed [8].

One such AAL cloud-based service-oriented architecture was elaborated during the development of the eWALL project [9]. eWALL is a platform providing dynamic environment for elderly patients with MCI and Chronic Obstructive Pulmonary Disease (COPD) for social interaction and continuous medical surveillance. The system offers personalized services such as daily activity monitoring, exercises, reminders and others.

The main contribution of this paper is the implementation in Sect. 2 of the Sleep Lifestyle Reasoner (SLR) which allows detection of minor or major deviations in the sleeping patterns in MCI patients indicating changes in their health status and being a good indication of the progression of their cognitive impairments. The output of the SLR is fed to the My Sleep Web Application described in Sect. 3. The added value of this personalized application is to support the primary user in the self-management of his condition and also to support the informal caregiver in providing insights on the sleeping behavior of the patient. It also provides recommendations to improve sleep hygiene and coach the users into a healthy sleeping behavior, based on their personal rhythms and problems.

## 2 Sleep Lifestyle Reasoner Description

A general description of the eWall architecture with all its components is given in [10]. The Lifestyle Reasoners (LR) within the eWALL are components which aim to predict behavior and to detect variations that might indicate a change in the user's health status. To do so, the LRs consume data from multiple sources and derive semantically meaningful patterns. The reasoner determines whether a variation falls within the expected thresholds, or employs more complex statistical methods to determine deviations and outliers.

Figure 1 illustrates the data flow regarding the sleep from sensor data acquisition to the SLR. The sensors existent in the user's room (microphone, accelerometer and bed pressure [11]) provide raw data to the Daily Functioning Service Brick (SB), which perform pre-processing algorithms as filtering. The Sleep Intelligent Decision Support System (IDSS) reasoner [11] then combines the data from the SB retrieved from several service endpoints and infer on the sleep period. The SLR runs once a day and, if new data is detected, creates updated averages of each one of the pre-defined parameters related to the sleeping pattern of the user. Averages are calculated using Linear Weighted Moving Average, giving bigger weight to more recent values. Outliers are filtered and not considered in the calculations.

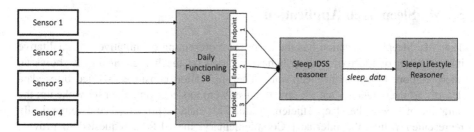

**Fig. 1.** Conceptualization of data flow from raw data acquired by sensors to *sleep_data* used by the lifestyle reasoner.

**Reasoner inputs:** The SLR gets data regarding the last night's sleep from the Sleep IDSS reasoner, which uses sleep data from a Fitbit tracker (a third party component, which delivers partially low level, partially high level reasoning - https://www.fitbit.com). Based on the data received, it infers the following parameters part of the *sleep_data*:

- bedOnTime: Time the user went to bed, in minutes since 0:00 of the day preceding the night.
- bedOffTime: Time the user got out of bed, in minutes since 0:00 of the day following the night.
- totalSleepTime: Total duration in minutes that the user was in bed during the night;
- frequencyWakingUp: Number of times that the user woke up during the night;
- sleepEfficiency: The sleep efficiency in percent.

**Reasoner outputs:** Weighted average in minutes of each parameter of sleep per day of the week till the current moment. The SLR has two JSON (JavaScript Object Notation) end-points. The "lastupdate" endpoint provides the date until which the reasoner has processed data for a specific user, and the "sleepweekpattern" provides the averaged sleep data for each day of the week for a specific user.

**Applications served:** The SLR generates data that is shown to the users by the following applications:

- My Sleep Application, providing patterns of sleep over time (e.g. usual time of going to sleep or usual sleep location);
- Personal Daily Support Service, whenever a notification should be provided to the user;
- Caregiver Application, whenever the caregiver should be informed about significant changes in the sleeping patterns of the primary user.

The SLR stores intermittent and processed results in the MongoDB database. By detecting deviations from normality, it supports MCI patients in the self-management of their condition. Also, as the sleeping period becomes, for example, more interrupted, the patient is alerted and it might lead him to be directed to a healthcare professional to control his condition. In order to meet the requirements of the MCI and COPD target groups, a set of different modules were defined. For each of these modules an appropriate scenario and their associated requirements are taken into account in the platform.

## 3  My Sleep Web Application

The "My Sleep" application has the purpose of presenting quantitative and qualitative interpretation of the user's sleep behavior based on the home sensing. It shows an interpretation of last night sleep data. The application consumes service brick data describing sleep events such as: time the user went to sleep; time the user woke up; the duration of sleep; the sleep efficiency, etc. This data is processed and semantically represented within the interface. Complementary, the SLR is requested to provide patterns of sleep behavior for the user and the information is displayed according to each sleep period described in the interface. These connections are depicted in Fig. 2.

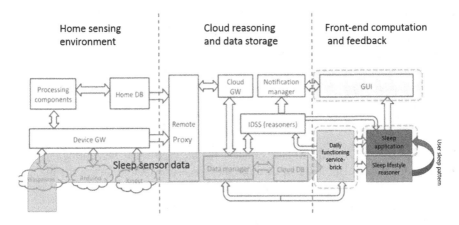

**Fig. 2.** Connection between the sleep application and the dependent eWALL components

Thus we present the user's last night behavior in the context of his routine behavior. Additionally, the application computes quality of sleep parameters, taking into account objective parameters according to medical norms in measuring quality of sleep. The sleep data can be visualized for one day at the time, or one week at the time. Figure 3(a) depicts the interface for the sleep application. The GUI was adapted to the recommendations which came out of the target group of eWALL users. On Fig. 3(a) and (b) is illustrated the summary of one night sleep expressed in 4 paragraphs. This implementation reduces considerably the information overload of the interface.

Sleep efficiency counts the proportion of time the user spends in bed with the intention of sleeping and the actual time spent sleeping. This measurement is expressed in percent.

Sleep time counts the total time in minutes the user has been sleeping (Fig. 4(a)). The number of awakenings during the sleep period is also important. The Fig. 4(b) shows the weekly overview of this measurement.

The outcomes from SLR output interpretation are represented through clear text in the daily view and color coded in the weekly view. The text is short and concise, eliminating the perception of "long boring read".

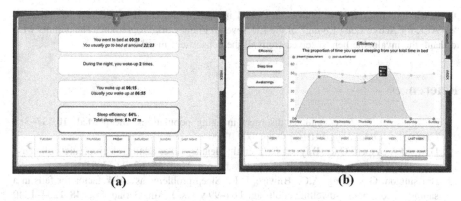

**Fig. 3.** The eWALL sleep application interface based on elderly user and expert user tests. (a) Depicts the daily sleep review. (b) Depicts weekly sleep efficiency view

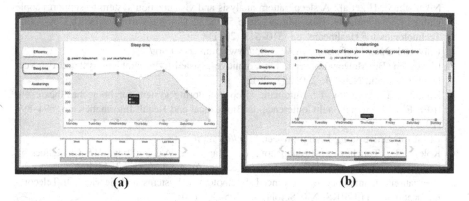

**Fig. 4.** (a) The eWALL sleep interface, depicting the sleep time panel, (b) depicting the awakening panel

## 4   Conclusion

In this paper we present an implementation of Sleep Lifestyle Reasoner allowing detection of changes in the sleeping patterns in MCI and COPD patients thus indicating changes in their health status. This information is useful for a sleep specialist who wants to check a patient's daily sleep pattern and also supports self-awareness about each individual sleeping patterns and create alerts whenever the sleeping behavior deviates from expected. The presented Web application offers to manage the user's profile and feedback for personalized recommendations on the basis of subject's interests, preferences and behavior. The application provides services according to the user's selected device (i.e., web interface, smartphone or tablet).

The design and implementation of most of eWALL software components including the lifestyle reasoners are operational and currently are in the phase of end-user testing.

**Acknowledgments.** This work was supported in part by the Grant Agreement No: 610658, "eWALL for Active Long Living" of the EU Seventh Framework Programme. The authors wish to thank the invaluable help received from all the consortium members.

# References

1. Ancoli-Israel, S.: Sleep and its disorders in aging populations. Sleep Med. **10**, S7–S11 (2009). https://doi.org/10.1016/j.sleep.2009.07.004
2. Dew, M.A., Hoch, C.C., Buysse, D.J., et al.: Healthy older adults' sleep predicts all-cause mortality at 4 to 19 years of follow-up. Psychosom. Med. **65**, 63–73 (2003)
3. Brassington, G.S., King, A.C., Bliwise, D.L.: Sleep problems as a risk factor for falls in a sample of community-dwelling adults aged 64–99 years. J. Am. Geriatr. Soc. **48**, 1234–1240 (2000)
4. da Silva, R.: Sleep disturbances and mild cognitive impairment: a review. Sleep Sci. **8**(1), 36–41 (2015). https://doi.org/10.1016/j.slsci.2015.02.001
5. Nikamalfard, H., et al.: A sleep pattern analysis and visualization system to support people with early dementia. In: Proceedings of the 5th ICST Conference on Pervasive Computing Technologies for Healthcare, pp. 510–513 (2011)
6. Universal Open Platform for AAL. http://www.universaal.org/
7. Li, R., Lu, B., McDonald-Maier, D.: Cognitive assisted living ambient system: a survey. Digit. Commun. Netw. **1**, 229–252 (2015)
8. Kitamura, K., Nemoto, T.: Automatic sleep monitoring system for home healthcare. In: IEEE-EMBS International Conference on Biomedical and Health Informatics, pp. 894–897 (2012)
9. Ewall for Active Long Living project. http://ewallproject.eu
10. Koleva, P., Tonchev, K., Balabanov, G., Manolova, A., Poulkov, V.: Challenges in designing and implementation of an effective Ambient Assisted Living system. In: International Conference on Advanced Technologies, Systems and Services in Telecommunications – TELSIKS, Niš, Serbia, pp. 305–308 (2015)
11. Tonchev, K., Koleva, P., Manolova, A., Tsenov, G., Poulkov, V.: Non-intrusive sleep analyzer for real time detection of sleep anomalies. In: 39th International Conference on Telecommunications and Signal Processing (TSP), Vienna, Austria (2016)

# Implementation of Daily Functioning and Habits Building Reasoner Part of AAL Architecture

Krasimir Tonchev[✉], Yuliyan Velchev, Pavlina Koleva,
Agata Manolova, Georgi Balabanov, and Vladimir Poulkov

Faculty of Telecommunications, Technical University of Sofia,
8 Kliment Ohridski blvd., Sofia 1000, Bulgaria
{k_tonchev, p_koleva, amanolova, grb, vkp}@tu-sofia.bg,
julian_s_velchev@abv.bg

**Abstract.** Individuals with Mild Cognitive Impairment (MCI) currently have few treatment options against memory loss. Solutions for caring for the elderly both efficacious and cost-effective are given by Ambient Assisted Living (AAL) architecture, promising the improvement of the Quality of Life (QoL) of patients. QoL factors that are important for the MCI patients include mood, pleasant engagements, physical mobility and health, and the ability to perform activities of daily living. In this paper, we propose a daily activity reasoner that monitors, measures and analyses in real time several everyday events for building habits diary and detecting abnormal behavior of the user, part of an effective AAL system. The proposed solution is based on a combination of mean shift clustering algorithm. The reasoner offers two primary functionalities: habits building and duration and frequency of events. The reasoner can predict the behavior and detect (slow or fast) changes that might indicate modification in the health status of the user.

**Keywords:** Daily activity monitoring · Habits measurement
Habit anomaly detection · GMM · K-means clustering

## 1 Introduction

Persons with mild cognitive impairment (MCI) experience declines in everyday functioning and cognitive performance greater than what is experienced in normal aging but less than that of dementia. Daily stress and daily memory complaints associated with cognitive deficits may contribute to greater psychological distress in the day-to-day experiences of people with MCI [1]. Supporting memory-related behavioral stability in MCI patients could help maintain their daily function and prolong the time before onset of dependency. According to [2] the decline in episodic memory is one of the defining features of MCI patients. Thus, early detection of cognitive dysfunction is of great importance in primary health care. In addition, assessment of everyday life activities should be performed in order to help medical personnel on when and how to intervene [3], and also for the affected to limit the effect of cognitive decline. According

© ICST Institute for Computer Sciences, Social Informatics and Telecommunications Engineering 2018
N. Oliver et al. (Eds.): MindCare 2016/Fabulous 2016/IIoT 2015, LNICST 207, pp. 113–118, 2018.
https://doi.org/10.1007/978-3-319-74935-8_16

to [4], individuals with MCI, their family members, and their care providers have all identified "quality of life" (QoL) as a central goal in the treatment of dementia and MCI. QoL factors include mood, engagement in pleasant activities, physical mobility and health, and the ability to perform activities of daily living. After identifying the essential features of good QoL, the key question is: how can we use this information to improve the daily l of individuals suffering from these conditions?

To date, interventions aimed at extending functional capacity in MCI have been pharmacologic in nature. While medications may produce delays in the progression of cognitive difficulties, individuals with MCI are also interested in additional activities they can do to maintain and improve their QoL by managing their memory loss [5]. One such solution is offered by Ambient Assisted Living (AAL), an emerging multi-disciplinary field aiming at providing an ecosystem of different types of sensors, computers, mobile devices, wireless networks and software applications for personal healthcare monitoring systems [6]. One such AAL cloud-based service-oriented architecture was elaborated during the development of the eWALL project [7].

The main contribution of this paper is to present a daily activity reasoner part of the eWALL architecture that monitors, measures and analyses in real time several events for building habits log/diary and detecting abnormal behavior of the user.

We describe the daily functioning reasoner, used to build and measure the habits of the user, relying on statistical approaches such as Gaussian Mixture Model (GMM) and K-means and mean shift (MS) clustering algorithms (Sect. 2). Discussion of the experimental results and proof of our theoretical assumption on artificial data and the output of the reasoner is done in Sect. 3.

## 2  Daily Functioning Lifestyle Reasoner Description

eWALL is a platform providing dynamic environment for elderly patients with MCI for social interaction and continuous medical surveillance. The system offers personalized services such as daily activity monitoring, suitable exercises, reminders and others.

Lifestyle Reasoners (LR) within the eWALL are components that process and store long term data that follows certain patterns defining the lifestyle of the user. The aim of these components is to predict behavior and to detect (slow or fast) changes that might indicate a change in the user's health status. To do so, the LRs consume data from multiple sources and derive semantically meaningful patterns. The data is processed, stored, and compared data stored in the cloud and the reasoner determines e.g. whether a variation falls within the expected thresholds, or employs more complex methods to determine deviation. The reasoners make decisions about the short-, medium-, or long-term past. The eWALL system has 10 LR: Vital Signs, Daily Physical Activity, Mood, Sleep, Daily Functioning, Home Environment, Calendar, Physical Trainer, Cognitive Training, and eWALL interaction.

A block diagram describing the algorithm for the Daily Functioning LR is presented in Fig. 1. The input of the algorithm is a list of pairs formed by timestamp and activity. Each timestamp marks the time that a change of activity (or "state") was detected, while the activity value itself represents the new activity that was detected. The algorithm has two branches working in parallel.

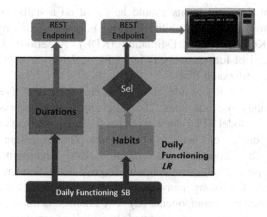

**Fig. 1.** Block diagram of Daily Functioning LR

The **Duration** branch collects all events for a monitoring period of 4 weeks. Using these events, duration of each one is calculated together with its statistical median value. The median value is preferred in order to avoid outliers which can introduce significant bias. The calculation of the averages is done only once a day. The monitoring period is tunable. The repetition of some of the daily functions is more important than their duration. Thus, this branch provides reasoning upon repetition of functions as well. Table 1 shows the types of activities and the performed reasoning.

**Table 1.** Types of daily activities

| Activity | Estimate | Reasoning |
|---|---|---|
| Entertaining | Mean value | Abnormal if more than 3 h per day |
| Showering | Median value | Abnormal if less than two times a week |
| Outdoors | Median value | Abnormal if less than two times a week |
| Socializing | Median value | Abnormal if less than two times a week |
| Sleeping | Mean value | Abnormal if less than 7 h per day |

The **Habits** branch involves more intelligent computing. It is using the low level information to build the habits of the user. Data for a monitoring period of 4 weeks is selected. It should be noted that the length of this period is a compromise between accuracy (larger interval) and responsiveness (smaller interval). The primary assumption is that the habits are repetitive activities, the start of each activity is within a certain time frame. Another assumption is that an activity can be repeated in the course of the week. All habits are built for a particular day of the week and are independent of the date or the day of the month. Once the habits are built, there is a further filtering by the block selection "Sel" (Fig. 1) based on the user's preferences about which of the habits he wants to be informed. The preferences are setup in the reasoner configuration. Every event received by the Habits reasoning is numbered and stamped with UTC time stamp in ms.

The analysis of the daily habits should be based on a statistical approach. One possibility is to estimate the Probability Density Function (PDF) by using a kernel method such as Kernel Density Estimation (KDE). A serious drawback of this approach is the need of further analysis in terms of detection of the modes and its parameters from the estimated PDF.

The other approach is to consider the task as clustering one. Every habit forms a cluster in the time and day of the week. The initial approach to address the clustering is the GMM [8]. In this model a PDF for a given habit can be approximated with arbitrary precision as superposition of Gaussian components. The estimation of parameters is typically done by the Expectation-Maximization (E-M) algorithm. The number of components (clusters) can be determined with Bayes Information Criterion (*BIC*). The optimal model is selected among many considering the insignificant decrease of *BIC* as a function of the number of components (*C*). The criterion is difficult to adjust, so the number of clusters is not always as expected. In addition sometimes a given cluster is incorrectly represented as a sum of two or more overlapped components. The GMM give an exact estimation of the mean and the standard deviation for a particular component, but any incorrect selection of *C* makes the data statistics hard for automated interpretation.

Since the GMM have not proved well in this particular application, the second technique that was used was the K-means clustering. The means and the standard deviations of the resulting clusters are close enough to those found with GMM and the robustness of the detection of the habits is superior to those of GMM estimation. The selection of the number of clusters is problematic since the algorithm is rough approximation of the GMM.

The MS clustering algorithm does not require a prior knowledge about the number of clusters and their shape. The calculation of the univariate kernel density estimate obtained with the radially symmetric kernels is described in [9]. Since the algorithm is intended to locate the modes in the histogram, it performs well in the described context. Using the priors (the number of elements in the cluster divided by the total number of observations) it is possible to retain only the significant clusters by appropriate threshold. Inappropriate bandwidth can cause modes to be merged, or generate additional "shallow" modes. A given habit can repeat few times daily and the histogram modes are spread apart from each other, so selecting lower values of the bandwidth and merging the adjacent clusters performed well in the experiments.

## 3    Experimental Results

For testing of the algorithms, the artificial data for a habit is generated as superposition of a uniformly distributed background of 30 events plus three components of ten events with normal distribution. The means are $20 \times 106$, $40 \times 106$ and $70 \times 106$ ms. The standard deviations are $0.6 \times 106$, $1.2.106$ and $2.4 \times 106$ ms. On Fig. 2(a) are illustrated the results of modes detection using GMM. The optimal number of clusters is chosen with *BIC* (Fig. 2(b)).

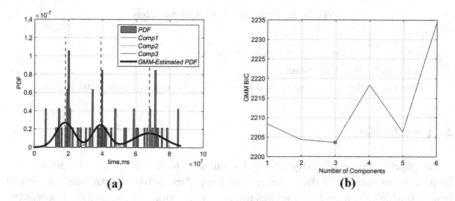

**Fig. 2.** (a) Daily habit estimation using GMM; (b) Number of components selection using *BIC*

For the same data a clustering using K-means is also performed (Fig. 3(a)). The best result in terms of background rejection and precision of the modes position is achieved with MS algorithm (Fig. 3(b)). The selected bandwidth is 5 × 106 ms.

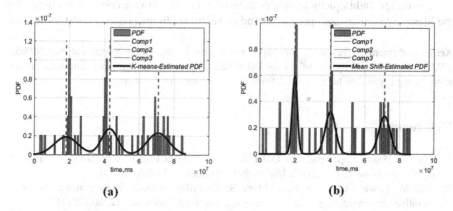

**Fig. 3.** (a) An example of daily habit estimation using K-means; (b) using mean shift

As can be seen from the figures, the clustering algorithm based on MS delivers promising results comparing to the others. This algorithm is working in a natural way with the data. The reasoner provides two endpoints of type GET returning data only upon request. Retrieving the habits is done by the method **habits** and its response is a list of the estimated habits. The parameters for each habit are described in Table 2.

Both methods don't have input parameters and the estimated values delivered by each are done based on an optimal time interval determined in the experiments.

Table 2. Parameters measured for habits

| Habits | |
| --- | --- |
| Habit | "Entertaining", "showering" etc. |
| Dayofweek | "Sunday", "monday" etc. |
| Timeofday | HH:mm:ss.SSSZ, local time zone of the user when the habit is done |

# 4 Conclusion

In this paper we present a daily activity LR intended to reason upon user's activities to be used as an automated diary. When analyzing these activities, patterns are formed based on which the reasoner estimates the user's behavior and assists him if necessary. The LR implements two primary functionalities: habits building and duration and frequency of events. It searches for repeating activities based on which it forms habits by taking into account the natural variations introduced by user's behavior. By reasoning upon the duration or frequency of different functionalities, for example, if the user is spending too much time watching TV, we can encourage him/her to do other activities and try to break down this habit.

The design and implementation of most of eWALL software components including the lifestyle reasoners are operational and currently are in the phase of end-user testing.

**Acknowledgments.** This work was supported in part by the Grant Agreement No: 610658, eWALL for Active Long Living" of the EU Seventh Framework Programme. The authors wish to thank the invaluable help received from all the consortium members.

# References

1. Hahn, E.: Daily Experiences of Older Adults with Mild Cognitive Impairment. Graduate Theses and Dissertation (2012). http://scholarcommons.usf.edu/etd/4060
2. Irish, M., Lawlor, B., Coen, R., O'Mara, S.: Everyday episodic memory in amnestic mild cognitive impairment: a preliminary investigation. BMC Neurosci. **12**, 80 (2011)
3. Johansson, M.: Cognitive impairment and its consequences in everyday life, Linköping University Medical Dissertation No. 1452 (2015)
4. Logsdon, R.G., McCurry, S.M., Teri, L.: Evidence-based interventions to improve quality of life for individuals with dementia. Alzheimers Care Today **8**(4), 309–318 (2007)
5. Greenaway, M., Hanna, S., Lepore, S., Smith, G.: A behavioral rehabilitation intervention for amnestic Mild Cognitive Impairment. Am. J. Alzheimers Dis. Other Demen. **23**(5), 451–461 (2008)
6. Universal Open Platform for AAL. http://www.universaal.org/
7. Ewall for Active Long Living project. http://ewallproject.eu
8. Aggarwal, C., Reddy, C.: Data Clustering: Algorithms and Applications. CRC Press, Boca Raton (2016)
9. Comaniciu, D., Meer, P.: Mean shift: a robust approach toward feature space analysis. IEEE Trans. Pattern Anal. Mach. Intell. **24**, 603–619 (2002)

# 5G-TCP: Enhanced Transport Protocol for Future Mobile Networks

Ivan Petrov[1($\boxtimes$)] and Toni Janevski[2]

[1] Sales Excellence Unit, Makedonski Telekom AD Skopje, Skopje, Macedonia
ivan.petrov@telekom.mk
[2] Faculty of Electrical Engineering and Information Technologies,
Saints Cyril and Methodius University, Skopje, Macedonia
tonij@feit.ukim.edu.mk

**Abstract.** Next generation of mobile networks are expected to assure super fast data transfer with very low delay. The initial 5G standardization is expected to be finalized around 2020. Enhanced mobile broadband with its corresponding demand of higher capacity and end user data rates represents the key driver of 5G network development. The transport protocols are directly correlated with the traffic rate, so they must be kept in the focus and should be properly designed. In this paper we present 5G-TCP as new applicable solution that improves the protocol performances over super fast mobile networks.

**Keywords:** 5G · Congestion control · Mobile networks · TCP
Transport protocol

## 1 Introduction

The next generation networks will have to assure radically lower cost and energy consumption per delivered bit. The network must offer higher data transfer rates in static and mobile mode of operation mainly because the conventional mobile broadband applications will demand higher capacity and higher end user data rates [1–4]. Next Generation (NGN) and Future Networks are all-IP networks, meaning that all data, control and signaling will be carried through IP communication, based on the Internet technologies from network protocol layer up to the application layer, with different heterogeneous access technologies on the lower two layers of the protocol stack [5]. In that manner 5G networks are expected to be all-IP with higher bit rates in the access and core parts, and delays less than 1 ms in the mobile terrestrial access part, that requires continuing work on the Internet protocol stack, which is consisted of IP (Internet Protocol) on the network layer and TCP (Transmission Control Protocol) and UDP (User Datagram Protocol) on the transport protocol layer. Our objective is to find generally applicable solutions that improve the protocol performance over high speed wireless and mobile access networks, while maintaining the performance over wired links in the mobile (NGN-based) core network. TCP is common denominator for many services, therefore by modifying TCP [7–14] the need for applying solutions locally can be reduced. We have designed and evaluated version of high speed TCP named as 5G-TCP, protocol that could be implemented in the future super fast networks.

© ICST Institute for Computer Sciences, Social Informatics and Telecommunications Engineering 2018
N. Oliver et al. (Eds.): MindCare 2016/Fabulous 2016/IIoT 2015, LNICST 207, pp. 119–125, 2018.
https://doi.org/10.1007/978-3-319-74935-8_17

The paper is organized as follows: Sect. 2 describes the basics of 5G-TCP, the simulation scenario and results are discussed in Sect. 3. Section 4 concludes the paper.

## 2 Description of 5G-TCP

It is interesting to notice that the function of parabola is generalized by rational normal curves which have coordinates $(x, x^2, x^3, ... x^n)$, standard parabola is obtained when $n = 2$ and the case when $n = 3$ is known as twisted cubic which is used as response function by TCP Cubic protocol [11]. In the theory of quadratic forms the parabola function represents the graph of the quadratic form $x^2$. The curves $y = x^p$ for other values of $p$ are referred as higher parabolas and are treated implicitly in the form $x^p = ky^q$. In accordance with this analysis we can find analogy with the standard TCP response function in time domain presented in the form as $2^{t/RTT}$, where RTT presents packet round trip time and $t$ is the current time or with the cubic function written as $x^3$ with the form $y = x^p$. It is native to conclude that several TCP protocols use parabola or higher parabola as common protocol response function. We have decided to use parabola function instead linear interpolation [8] at log log scale in order to define $w(p)$. If we put series of circles in the same plane as the curve, by keeping one of the segments constant we can construct parabola. At Fig. 1 is presented construction of parabola with help of series of tangent circles passing through the point S. The segment SA is kept constant during the construction. The fixed horizontal line at A constructs geometric means between SA (constant) and the series of segments AT, AU, AV. These segments are plotted against the series of geometric means AX, AY, AZ to give the points A, B, C, D all of which lie along the parabola. The vertical distances of the points (B, C and D) form A are proportional to the square on their horizontal distances.

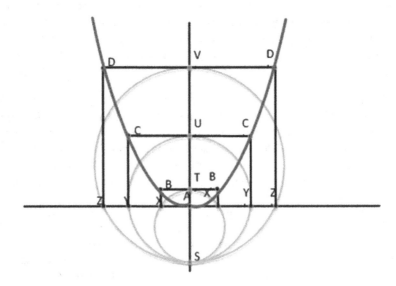

**Fig. 1.** Design of parabola with help of circles

Knowing how to construct parabola with help of this method we came to idea to present the TCP response function in the same manner. We have analyzed HSTCP [8] in details and have decided instead to use equation of line at log log scale for known two points defined with congestion window value (cwnd, w) and packet drop rate (p) to construct function of parabola uniquely defined with known three points.

We have named this protocol 5G-TCP and have decided to keep the predefined switch point used by HSTCP defined with w = 38 and p = $10^{-3}$. In order to construct parabola we have used the following points w1 = 8300 pkt and p1 = $10^{-4}$ (corresponds at speed of 1 Gbps), w2 = 830000 pkt and p2 = $10^{-7}$ (corresponds at speed of 100 Gbps), w3 = 3330000 and p3 = $10^{-12}$ (corresponds at speed of 400 Gbps). These points are chosen because 1 Gbps is expected to be common data transfer rate of 5G mobile networks, 100 Gbps is expected to be backhaul link speed and 400 Gbps is the theoretical speed of optical link defined with IEEE P802.3bs standard. If we have this standardization in mind then we can decade to use future 5G network packet loss probability values and data rates to define our switch points.

Recall that suggested bit error probabilities are real if we use 1500 byte packets. We have tried with these predefined points to calculate the constant distance SA and to use it to plot the parabola function with help of one point tangent circles. Knowing that the process can be translated in algorithm that can calculate next cwnd value was promising until we found that with this set of points we obtain different SA values mainly because the chosen points define the function f1 presented at Fig. 2 which does not corresponds with the one presented at Fig. 1. After we have obtained the result we decided to use the standard parabola equation to define f1 graphically and analytical with help of (1) or (2).

$$y = ax^2 + bx + c \qquad (1)$$

$$\log(w) = a(\log(p))^2 + b\log(p) + c \qquad (2)$$

y represents log (cwnd) and x is written as log(p). For known three points (defined with w, p; w2, p2 (100 Gbps) and w3, p3 (400 Gbps)) we can unique define function of parabola and if we solve the system of three equations we will define the values of a, b and c. Following values were calculated a = −0.108, b = −2.17 and c = −3.96 which define the function f1 presented at Fig. 2 We have calculated the values of a = −0.41, b = −5.21 and c = −10.47, case when the points of interest are (w, p), (w1, p1) and (w2, p2) that construct f2 which cuts f1 at point B.

Obtained functions f1 and f2 are not adequate to be used mainly because for very small values of p (p < $10^{-12}$ case when f1 is used and p < $10^{-7}$ case when f2 is used) cwnd value starts to drop which is not desired. We have decided to solve the system of equations once more but this time for points that correspond at speed of 5 Mbps when p = $10^{-3}$, 10 Mbps when p = $10^{-4}$ and 100 Mbps with p = $10^{-5}$. Following parameter values were calculated a = 0.325, b = 1.92, c = 4.42 which define the third function f3 presented at Fig. 2. f3 cuts f1 in point A when cwnd corresponds at rate of 53 Gbps (w4) and p4 = $10^{-6.58}$. We found that f3 can be constructed and plotted with help of the method described above. We have plotted two additional functions with help of the equation of line, case when cwnd corresponds at rate of 400 Gbps, f4 and f5 which cut f1 at different p values, the first one in point C (p5 = $10^{-8}$)and the other one in point D (p6 = $10^{-12}$).

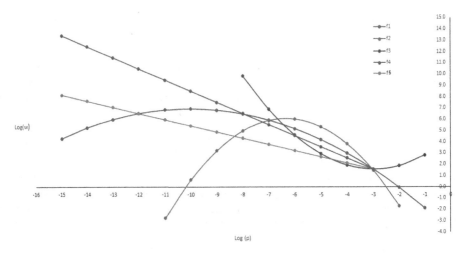

**Fig. 2.** Graphical presentation of f1, f2, f3, f4, f5

From Fig. 2 we conclude that the response function choice can be improved. Final 5G-TCP response function is defined with f3 when w < cwnd < w4 and p4 < p < p, when w4 < cwnd < w5 and p5 < p < p4 the protocol will use f1 as a response function. For values larger than w5 or when p is smaller or equal than p5 the protocol will use the function f4. The equation of line can be easily transformed from log domain but this does not stand for the equation of parabola. It is important to note that this protocol uses different response functions for low and high speed data rates which make it TCP friendly. Standard parabola is defined with:

$$x^2 = ky \tag{3}$$

or with

$$x^2 = y \tag{4}$$

In log log scale we will have

$$\log(p)^2 = \log(w) \tag{5}$$

$$\log(p) = \frac{\log(w)}{\log(p)} \equiv \log_p(w) \tag{6}$$

$$w = p^{\log(p)} \tag{7}$$

In the case when Eq. (3) is used we will have

$$w = p^{\log(p)^{\frac{1}{k}}} \tag{8}$$

If we plot Eq. (7) we will obtain the representation at Fig. 3 from where it is clear that for very small values of p, w enlarges its value and asymptotically nears the y axis. We can say that the Eqs. (7) and (8) define the 5G-TCP response function α is calculated as in [8], while β can be described with parabola function passing through 0.1 when w = 3330000, p = $10^{-12}$; 0.5 when w = 38 and p = $10^{-3}$; 0.4 when w = 833 pkt (100 Mbps).

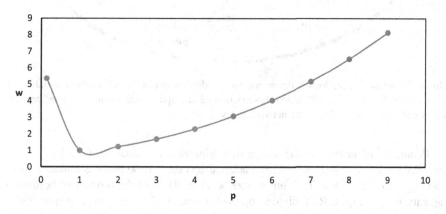

**Fig. 3.** Graphical presentation of Eq. (7)

For cwnd values larger that 3330000 pkt β will be calculated according equation of line defined with given two points w and w3.

$$\beta(w) = (0.1 - 0.5)\frac{\log(w) - \log(38)}{\log(3330000) - \log(38)} + 0.5 \tag{9}$$

Following values were calculated for a = −.003, b = −0.05 and c = 0.59. We will obtain similar results if we use Eq. (9) to calculate β(w). It is important to note that variance during β(w) calculation is noticed for lower cwnd values so we advice parabola function to be used in that case.

## 3   Simulation Scenario

The simulation scenario is presented at Fig. 4, analysis is conducted in order to justify the 5G-TCP design. We use the network simulator (ns2) upgraded with 5G-TCP module. At Fig. 6 we have presented communication of mobile terminal with base station and backhaul high speed link connected with adequate network gateway.

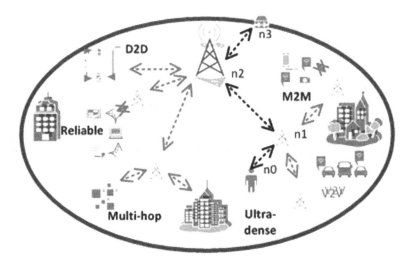

**Fig. 4.** Simulation scenario. We define wireless medium between n0 and micro base station n1. n1 is wirelessly connected with macro base station n2 and optical link n2–n3 is defined between the macro base station n2 and the network gateway n3

Parameter of interest is the congestion window size variation. Cwnd is directly related with the achieved throughput. Packet size is set at 1500 bytes. Simulation run is 2000 s. Buffers are Drop Tail; buffer size is set at 100% of the product of bottleneck capacity by the largest RTT divided by packet size. The result is presented at Fig. 5. Where we present w as a function of time. It can be noticed that Reno protocol has smallest window growth which directly impacts the throughput that can be achieved when this protocol is used. HSTCP cwnd change compared with Reno is more than

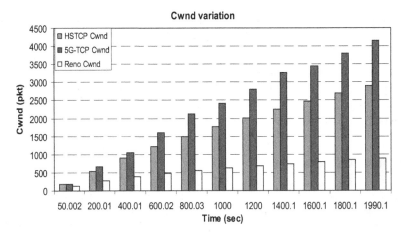

**Fig. 5.** Congestion window (cwnd) change for Gbps mobile connections with adequate buffer sizes of 8300, 83000 and 166000 packets.

doubled over the time. 5G-TCP presents improved results when compared with HSTCP for sessions longer than 50 s. As we have described in the previous section 5G-TCP employs fast growing function that makes it superior.

# 4   Conclusion

In this paper we have presented new high speed TCP algorithm with help of detail analysis of HSTCP design. Increased friendliness and higher data rates are achieved when 5G-TCP is employed in predefined simulation environment. The protocol is defined to be used in the future 5G data networks regardless of the engaged MAC Layer. It is defined with several response functions for variety of speeds up to 400 Gbps. For sure the development of high speed protocols that will follow the 5G network capacity is essential in order the end user to experience the network capacity benefit. 5G-TCP represents high speed protocol that uses parabola in order to define the protocol response function and the calculation of $\beta(w)$ parameter. 5G-TCP should provide efficient usage of the network capacity up to speed of 400 Gbps.

# References

1. Duke, M., Braden, R., Eddy, W., Blanton, E., Zimmermann, A.: A roadmap for Transmission Control Protocol (TCP). Internet Engineering Task Force (IETF), RFC7414, February 2015
2. Janevski, T.: Internet Technologies for Fixed and Mobile Networks. Artech House, USA (2015)
3. Rodriguez, J.: Fundamentals of 5G Mobile Networks. Wiley, UK (2015)
4. Ge, X., Cheng, H., Guizani, M., Han, T.: 5G wireless backhaul networks: challenges and research advances. IEEE Netw. **28**(6), 6–11 (2014)
5. Janevski, T.: NGN Architectures, Protocols, and Services. Wiley, UK (2014)
6. Gunduz, D., Stamatiou, K., Michelusi, N., Zorzi, M.: Designing intelligent energy harvesting communication systems. IEEE Commun. Mag. **52**(1), 210–216 (2014)
7. Kelly, T.: Scalable TCP: improving performance in highspeed wide area networks. Comput. Commun. Rev. **32**(2), April 2003
8. Floyd, S.: HighSpeed TCP for large congestion windows. RFC 3649 (2003)
9. Xu, L., Harfoush, K., Rhee, I.: Binary increase congestion control for fast, long distance networks. In: Proceedings of the IEEE INFOCOM, vol. 4, pp. 2514–2524, March 2004
10. Leith, D.: H-TCP: TCP congestion control for high bandwidth-delay product paths. IETF Internet Draft (2008). http://tools.ietf.org/html/draftleith-tcp-htcp-06
11. Rhee, I., Xu, L.: CUBIC: a new TCP-friendly high-speed TCP variant. SIGOPS Oper. Syst. Rev. **42**(5), 64–74 (2008)
12. Marfia, G., Palazzi, C., Pau, G., Gerla, M., Sanadidi, M., Roccetti, M.: TCP Libra: Exploring RTT-Fairness for TCP. UCLA Computer Science Department, Technical Report UCLA-CSD TR-050037 (2005)
13. Caini, C., Firrincieli, R.: TCP Hybla: a TCP enhancement for heterogeneous networks. Int. J. Satell. Commun. Network. **22**, 547–566 (2004)
14. Baiocchi, A., Castellani, A.P., Vacirca, F.: YeAH-TCP: yet another highspeed TCP. In: Proceedings of the PFLDnet, ISI, Marina Del Rey (Los Angeles), California, February 2007

# Monitoring the Black Sea Region Using Satellite Earth Observation and Ground Telemetry

George Suciu[1,2(✉)], Octavian Fratu[1], Victor Suciu[2],
and Iulian Grigore[2]

[1] Telecommunications Department, University Politehnica of Bucharest,
Iuliu Maniu, 1-3, 061071 Bucharest, Romania
george.suciu@radio.pub.ro, ofratu@elcom.pub.ro
[2] R&D Department, Beia Consult International,
Str. Peroni, 12, 041386 Bucharest, Romania
{george,victor.suciu,iulian.grigore}@beia.ro

**Abstract.** The Black Sea region is affected by important environmental transformations and EO (Earth Observation) is considered a new way to monitor and, possibly, solve some of its critical issues. The ecological alterations, essentially caused by anthropogenic factors, are the main cause of many transformations such as the ecosystem changes, coastal erosion or pollution that affects water quality. The purpose of this paper is to present the environmental measurements performed with ground telemetry systems near the Black Sea coast in the Danube Delta and the fusion of sensor data with datasets from EO satellite applications. We present the BEIA telemetry system that has been installed and is further being developed for the National Administration "Romanian Waters" (ANAR), an automatic system able to continuously monitor the level and water temperature along the Danube, Danube Delta and some of its tributary rivers. Furthermore, we demonstrate how big data processing software can be used for extracting non-trivial correlations from telemetry and EO data. This paper is a general overview of the results for telemetry and EO integration in the Black Sea and the Danube region and could support ESA (European Space Agency) in defining future investments in EO research and development activities to foster EO innovation in the region.

**Keywords:** Ground telemetry · Satellite observation · Black Sea
Danube river · Water quality

## 1 Introduction

The Black Sea has been affected by significant ecological alterations caused by the anthropogenic factors. The major issues affecting the environmental state of Black Sea are pollution, loss of biodiversity and coastal degradation [1]. Scientists have identified several serious problems for the Black Sea associated with various types of pollution. One of them is the eutrophication phenomenon of the sea by nutrients which are compounds of nitrogen and phosphorus, as a result of pollution from domestic,

© ICST Institute for Computer Sciences, Social Informatics and Telecommunications Engineering 2018
N. Oliver et al. (Eds.): MindCare 2016/Fabulous 2016/IIoT 2015, LNICST 207, pp. 126–132, 2018.
https://doi.org/10.1007/978-3-319-74935-8_18

agricultural and industrial sources [2]. Another type of pollution is caused by oil spills. Oil interacts with the marine environment as a result of operational or accidental discharges from vessels, as well as through insufficiently treated wastewaters from land based sources [1]. Heavy metals such as cadmium, copper, chromium and lead are usually associated with waste from the heavy industry and ash remaining from burning coal usually used for generating electricity. Furthermore, pesticides enter the sea mostly through rivers and streams due to agriculture [2]. Another major problem is the discharge of insufficiently treated sewage waters, which leads to microbiological contamination and poses a threat to public health. Radioactive substances have been introduced to the Black Sea in small quantities from nuclear power plants and in more significant amounts after the nuclear power plant disaster from Chernobyl which occurred in 1986 [3]. An unusual form of pollution from ships is the introduction of exotic species, mostly through exchange of ballast waters or other wastewaters. The final major type of problematic pollutants is solid waste, dumped into the sea from ships and some coastal towns [4]. In that situation, Earth Observation (EO) could provide an opportunity for applications, innovative science and information services to deal with these problems.

The paper is organized as follows: Section 2 presents related work in the field of telemetry. Section 3 presents the proposed solution for tele-monitoring while Sect. 4 analyses the obtained results. Finally, Sect. 5 draws the conclusion and envisions future research directions.

## 2 Related Work

Through the MarineGeoHazard [5] project, implemented by Romania and Bulgaria, the main focus is to manage natural hazards at the Black Sea and the risks associated with their effects in trans-border area of the Romanian-Bulgarian coast. Also, there was implemented a rapid alert system in real time for the Black Sea, "Black Sea Security System", implemented in both Romania and Bulgaria, capable of delivering in continuous mode to the authorities of the two countries specific information which may lay at the basis of the decision-making [6].

Furthermore, the EUXINUS [7] project developed the first complex system for monitoring-alarm in real time to the marine hazards, with the risk to the coastal zone of Romania. The network is composed of three buoys EuxRO1, EuxRO2, EuxRO3 which are located on the Romanian continental plateau, in the territorial waters of Romania. For example, Surface Buoy (SRB) with the following features were deployed: solar recharging for the batteries, the management of the electrical supply of the base station, shiftable communications satellite/radio, data acquisition with the integrated management system, the remote control and communication in real time radio/satellite, weather sensors, active and passive radar, optical signals, acoustic output for the management of the communication and transmission of the data with installed submarine equipment. Furthermore, multiparametric wells were fixed at 5 m depth which includes sensors for: current, conductivity, temperature, pressure, oxygen, turbidity, chlorophyll and tsunamometer which is mounted on the bottom of the sea near the buoy [8]. It includes an anchoring system, a battery system for the supply of the sensors and a tsunamometer positioned on the bottom of the sea with acoustic modem for bidirectional communication with the surface buoy with remote triggering system. In [9] the water quality was monitored in the Black Sea region based on two characteristics: ecological status and chemical status. Furthermore, the Romanian National Center for Monitoring and Alarming to Natural Marine Hazards presented in [10] hardware devices used for the evaluation of the impact of the marine geohazards by providing maps in a standard GIS format.

## 3  Proposed Solution

For the tele-monitoring of the water level and the temperature in the Black Sea region along the Danube and some of its tributary rivers, an automatic system was installed under a continuous development for the ANAR ("Administratia Nationala Apele Romane") [11]. This system consists of some central elements, such as the Data Concentrator (Gateway) and the data presentation server. Data concentrator (Gateway) performs communication with the remote telemetry units (RTUs) and also allows the configuration and management of all RTUs and sensors. The data is presented in various formats so the users with the rights to change it could choose the one who suits their needs. Data processed by the presentation server are continuously and automatically exported towards ANAR's central data and dispatcher systems.

The monitoring system with GPRS has the schematic flow of data as presented in Fig. 1.

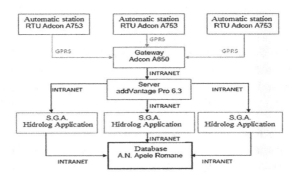

**Fig. 1.** Schematic flow of data

The RTU and the telemonitoring are powered by a solar panel, while a combo sensor for air temperature and relative humidity can be found at the recently installed ones. All sensors attached to a certain RTU are powered and read during short periodic time intervals. At every 15 min, the RTU computes from periodic measurement results an average value. At every hour, the 4 average values for every of the monitored parameters is sent by the RTU to the A850 central gateway. At the ANAR headquarters, the installation consists of a gateway (Adcon A850) and the application server addVantage Pro 6.3 which transfers data from the gateway and has the following functions: data visualization tools, basic editing tools data and it has a module that allows data export in different file formats.

## 4    Results

In this section we present and evaluate the results of measurements performed with water quality sensors, for sediments and results of satellite observation of the Black Sea region.

The data are high-resolution radar images obtained by the radars onboard Envisat satellite (till the spring of 2012) and Sentinel-1, starting from October 2014 [11]. Figure 2 shows the cumulative map of oil-containing spills. These pollution events are caused by spillages of oil-containing waters from moving ships. Also near the major ports of Bulgaria, Turkey, Romania and Ukraine a large amount of spills is observed near oil loading terminals.

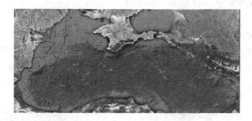

**Fig. 2.** Map of oil spills on the Black Sea surface revealed from the satellite radar imagery

In Fig. 3 we present some numerical data on oil spills in the Black Sea aquatic area. From the charts it can be seen that over 40% of spills detected in radar images do not exceed 1 km$^2$ and polluted areas in 80% of events are less than 5 km$^2$. However the ships discharges wastewaters several times while they are under way and under the influence of the wind and waves, the film spreads over the sea surface covering large areas. During warm season are registered the larger numbers of spills. As an explanation, the better weather conditions are favorable for recognition of spills in satellite radar images.

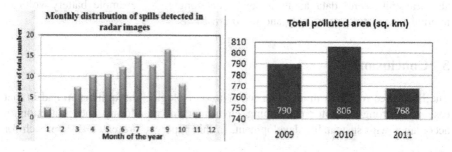

**Fig. 3.** Statistic data for oil spills

Furthermore, Fig. 4 provides a representation of the oil pollution on the Black Sea and can specify that pollution is produced by different sources as oil spills and under the influence of the wind and waves, the film spreads over the sea surface covering large areas.

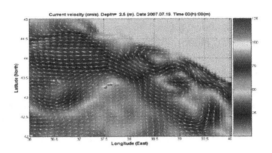

**Fig. 4.** Surface currents field by Black Sea operational model output. Predicted daily shift of the oil spill from red to yellow (Color figure online)

In Fig. 5 we present the observation of a great mass of water at the monitoring station Unirea (close to Cernavoda), with level changes slower than those at a monitoring station situated about 300 km upstream, at Bechet. Evolutions at Unirea are lagging behind evolutions at Bechet with something like 2–3 days.

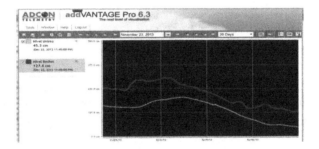

**Fig. 5.** Water level on the Danube measured using the ground telemetry system

Besides accurately reading and transmitting data from attached sensors, the RTUs also transmit useful data about its own functioning, for example battery voltage, internal temperature, data delay and radio error rate.

## 5 Conclusions

The Black Sea region is in an advanced state of ecological disequilibrium and in that case is a strong need for developing environmental monitoring and protection in accordance with sustainable development. In this paper we presented an approach for using data from Satellite Earth Observation and Ground Telemetry for monitoring environmental parameters. The performed observations have demonstrated a clear necessity to implement telemetry monitoring on Delta, Danube and Black Sea waters, so the proposed system, which provides water level monitoring, has potential to be extend in order to assess further water parameters.

As future work we will analyze satellite and ground telemetry data to cover further requirements for water quality monitoring, such as pH, dissolved, algae, oxygen and turbidity.

**Acknowledgments.** The work has been supported in part by UEFISCDI Romania under grants no. 20/2012 "Scalable Radio Transceiver for Instrumental Wireless Sensor Networks - SaRaT-IWSN", MobiWay, EV-BAT, CarbaDetect, and funded in part by grant no. 262EU/2013 "eWALL" support project, grant no. 337E/2014 "Accelerate" project, by European Commission by FP7 IP project no. 610658/2013 "eWALL for Active Long Living - eWALL" and European Union's Horizon 2020 research and innovation program under grant agreement No. 643963 (SWITCH project).

# References

1. Tuncer, G., Karakas, T., Balkas, T.I., Gökçay, C.F., Aygnn, S., Yurteri, C., Tuncel, G.: Land-based sources of pollution along the Black Sea coast of Turkey: concentrations and annual loads to the Black Sea. Mar. Pollut. Bull. **36**(6), 409–423 (1998)
2. Vasilescu, A., Suciu, G., Suciu, V.: Monitoring the danube with adcon telemetry equipment– a case study for OTT hydromet and rowater company. In: Conference Proceedings of 2nd International Conference on "Water Resources and Wetlands" -WATER 2014, pp. 221–230 (2014)
3. Gulin, S.B., Egorov, V.N., Duka, M.S., Sidorov, I.G., Proskurnin, V.Y., Mirzoyeva, N.Y., Bey, O.N., Gulina, L.V.: Deep-water profiling of 137Cs and 90Sr in the Black Sea: a further insight into dynamics of the post-chernobyl radioactive contamination. J. Radioanal. Nucl. Chem. **304**(2), 779–783 (2015)
4. Galatchi, L.D.: The Romanian national accidental and intentional polluted water management system. In: Dura, G., Kambourova, V., Simeonova, F. (eds.) Management of Intentional and Accidental Water Pollution, pp. 181–184. Springer, Netherlands (2006). https://doi.org/10.1007/1-4020-4800-9_16
5. Oaie, G., Secrieru, D., Seghedi, A., Ioane, D., Diaconescu, M.: Preliminary assessment of the tsunami hazard for the Romanian Black Sea area: historical and paleotsunami data. In: Geosciences, pp. 300–302 (2006)
6. Dobrev, N.D., Dimitrov, O.V., Nikolov, G.P., Kostov, K.S.: The first steps for a joint Romanian-Bulgarian regional early-warning system for marine geohazards. In: 8th Congress of the Balkan Geophysical Society (2015)
7. Radulescu, V., Oaie, G., Samoila, I.: EUXINUS-black sea security system-two years of operation. In: 8th Congress of the Balkan Geophysical Society (2015)
8. Zaytsev, A., Pelinovsky, E., Yalciner, A., Ionescu, C., Iren, M.: Assessment of tsunami hazard for western coast of the Black sea. In: EGU General Assembly Conference Abstracts, vol. 17, p. 10262 (2015)

9. Tuchiu, E., David, A.M.: The analysis of the anthropogenic pressures and their impacts of the Danube River in lower sector. In: Conference Proceedings Water Resources and Wetlands

10. Partheniu, R., Ionescu, C., Constantin, A., Moldovan, I., Diaconescu, M., Marmureanu, A., Radulian, M., Toader, V.: Tsunamis hazard assessment and monitoring for the Back Sea area. In: EGU General Assembly Conference Abstracts, vol. 18, p. 6703 (2016)

11. Ochian, A., Suciu, G., Fratu, O., Suciu, V.: Big data search for environmental telemetry. In: IEEE International Black Sea Conference on Communications and Networking (Black-SeaCom), pp. 182–184 (2014)

# Multi-microphone Noise Reduction System Integrating Nonlinear Multi-band Spectral Subtraction

Radu Mihnea Udrea, Claudia Cristina Oprea$^{(\boxtimes)}$, and Cristian Stanciu

Telecommunication Department, University Politehnica of Bucharest,
Iuliu Maniu 1-3, 061071 Bucharest, Romania
{mihnea, cristina, cristian}@comm.pub.ro

**Abstract.** This paper presents a robust system to improve speech signals processed by communication systems. The system includes multi-microphone techniques, for which both spectral and spatial characteristics of the signal sources can be used. Also a spectral subtraction algorithm for noise reduction is integrated into the system. The modified spectral subtraction method takes into account the non-uniform effect of colored noise on the speech spectrum and improves the multi-microphone noise filtering.

**Keywords:** Speech enhancement · Multi-microphone noise reduction

## 1 Introduction

Speech signal is often accompanied by environmental noise. There are several negative effects during processing the degraded speech for applications such as: automobile speech communication systems, voice recognition systems, speech recognition, speaker authentication.

Improvement techniques can be classified as a single channel, dual-channel and multiple channel speech enhancement techniques. Techniques to improve single channel speech [1] apply to situations in which only one microphone is available. In dual channel enhancement techniques, a reference signal for the noise is available and therefore adaptive noise cancellation technique can be applied. Multiple channel techniques use microphone array [2] and take advantage of the availability of multiple signal inputs to our system to make possible to use the phase alignment to reject unwanted noise components [3]. Beamforming is a multi-microphone signal processing technique that achieves a more directional pattern than what could be obtained with only one microphone.

The spatial-filter-based beamformers have been developed for narrow-band signals [4], which can be characterized by a single frequency. For the speech signal, which has a broadband frequency domain, the beamformers will not yield the same model for different frequencies and the beamwidth decreases as frequency increases. If we use such a beamformer when the steering direction is different from the incident angle of the source, the source signal will be low-pass filtered. In addition, the noise coming

© ICST Institute for Computer Sciences, Social Informatics and Telecommunications Engineering 2018
N. Oliver et al. (Eds.): MindCare 2016/Fabulous 2016/IIoT 2015, LNICST 207, pp. 133–138, 2018.
https://doi.org/10.1007/978-3-319-74935-8_19

from another direction, will not be attenuated evenly across its entire spectrum, resulting in some disturbing artifacts in the output array.

In this paper we propose integrating a nonlinear multi-band spectral subtraction noise reduction method into the beamforming system. The multi-band spectral subtraction applies different subtraction factors depending on the SNR in each frequency band. Because the beamformer will not attenuate uniformly the noise over entire spectrum, the proposed method will compensate this non-uniformity. The simulations are performed using a car environment with engine noise background.

## 2 Microphone Array Processing

Consider an array of $M$ microphones in a reverberant and acoustical noisy environment. The $i^{th}$ microphone output can be expressed as [2]:

$$y_i(n) = s(n) * h_i(n) \tag{1}$$

where $s(n)$ represents the clean speech signal, $h_i(n)$ denotes the impulse response between the speech source and the $i^{th}$ microphone and * denotes convolution.

There are fixed and adaptive beamforming systems. Fixed beamformer focus on source direction and therefore captures less noise and reverberation arrive from a different direction than the source. Adaptive beamformer provides better noise reduction, but it doesn't reduce the reverberation on other directions.

In a conventional delay-and-sum beamformer (DSB), $y_i(n)$ is first shifted by a time-delay $n_i$ and then scaled by a corresponding weight $w_i$. The resulting delayed and scaled signals from all microphones are then summed to produce the beamformer output $z(n)$:

$$z(n) = s(n) * g(n) \tag{2}$$

where

$$g(n) = \sum_{i=1}^{M} w_i h_i(n - n_i) \tag{3}$$

The purpose of the delays $n_i$ is to time-align the direct path components of the impulse responses $h_i(n)$ so as to steer the beamformer in the direction of the desired speech source. This way, the direct-path signals are phase-aligned and reinforced while echoes apart from the steering direction are attenuated.

The fixed spatial-filter beamformer directivity pattern will have a main lobe on the direction of the source speech signal and several secondary lobes. The characteristic changes depending of the frequency as shown in Fig. 1.

For the speech signal, which has a broadband frequency domain, such beamformers will not offer the same filtering model for different frequencies. As seen in Fig. 1 the beamwidth decreases as frequency increases. Therefore, the source signal will be low-pass filtered and the noise coming from another direction will not be attenuated evenly across its entire spectrum, resulting in some disturbing artifacts in the output array.

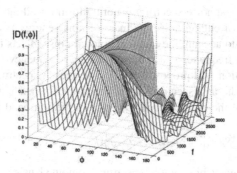

**Fig. 1.** The directivity characteristic of a fixed DS beamformer depending on the steering angle $\phi$ and frequency $f$.

## 3   The Spectral Subtraction Method

The basic assumption of the method is treating the noise as uncorrelated additive noise. Assume that a speech signal $s(n)$ has been degraded by the uncorrelated additive noise signal $d(n)$:

$$y(n) = s(n) + d(n) \tag{4}$$

Short time power spectrum of the noisy speech can be approximated by:

$$|Y(k)|^2 \approx |S(k)|^2 + |D(k)|^2 \tag{5}$$

The power spectral subtraction estimator results by replacing noise square-magnitude $|D(k)|^2$ with its average value taken during non-speech activity period.

$$\hat{\sigma}_d^2(k) \simeq E\left\{|D(k)|^2\right\} \tag{6}$$

Berouti [1] proposed an important variation of spectral subtraction for reduction of residual musical noise. An overestimate of the noise power spectrum is subtracted and the resulted spectrum is limited from going below a preset minimum level (spectral floor). The proposed algorithm could be expressed as:

$$|\hat{S}(k)|^2 = \begin{cases} |Y(k)|^2 - \alpha \cdot \hat{\sigma}_d^2(k), & \text{if } |\hat{S}(k)|^2 > \beta \cdot \hat{\sigma}_d^2(k) \\ \beta \cdot \hat{\sigma}_d^2(k), & \text{otherwise} \end{cases} \tag{7}$$

where $\alpha$ is the over-subtraction factor and $\beta$ is the spectral floor parameter.

To reduce the speech distortion caused by large values of $\alpha$, its value is adapted from frame to frame [5]. The basic idea is to take into account that the subtraction process must depend on the segmental noisy signal to noise ratio (NSNR) of the frame, in order to apply less subtraction with high NSNRs and vice versa.

In real environments, noise spectrum is not uniform for all the frequencies [6]. For example, in the case of engine noise the most of noise energy is concentrated in low frequency. To take into account the fact that colored noise affects the speech spectrum differently at various frequencies, a multi-band linear frequency spacing approach to spectral over-subtraction was proposed in [7]. The speech spectrum is divided into N non-overlapping bands, and spectral subtraction is performed independently in each band. The estimate of the clean speech spectrum in the $i$-th band is obtained by:

$$\left|\hat{S}_i(k)\right|^2 = |Y_i(k)|^2 - \alpha_i \cdot \hat{\sigma}_d^2(k), \quad v_i < k < v_{i+1} \tag{8}$$

where $k$ is the frequency bin for the spectrum computed using the discrete Fourier transform, $v_i$ and $v_{i+1}$ are the beginning and ending frequency bins of the $i$-th frequency band and $\alpha_i$ is the over-subtraction factor of the $i$-th band.

The over-subtraction factor $\alpha_i$ can be calculated as:

$$\alpha_i = \begin{cases} 1 & \gamma_i \geq 20\,\text{dB} \\ \alpha_0 - \frac{3}{20}\gamma_i & -5\,\text{dB} \leq \gamma_i \leq 20\,\text{dB} \\ 4.75 & \gamma_i \leq -5\,\text{dB} \end{cases} \tag{9}$$

where $\alpha_0 = 4$ and the aposteriori NSNR $\gamma_i$ of the $i$-th frequency band is:

$$\gamma_i(dB) = 10\log_{10} \frac{\sum\limits_{k=w_i}^{w_{i+1}} |X_i(k)|^2}{\sum\limits_{k=w_i}^{w_{i+1}} \hat{\sigma}_d^2(k)^2} \tag{10}$$

A nonlinear frequency spacing approach for multi-band over-subtraction factor estimation was proposed in [7] based on the fact that human ear sensibility varies nonlinear in frequency spectrum. A perceptual spectral estimation of critical bandwidth was involved, denoting the noise bandwidth limit at which the detection threshold of the signal (tone) ceased to increase. The noise power within the same critical band with the signal is then equal to the product of the measured power spectral density and the critical bandwidth of the band in question.

## 4    Implementation and Experimental Results

We simulate a microphone array configuration to enhance the speech signal inside an automobile. We considered a linear array with a variable number of 2 to 6 microphones equally spaced at a distance of 0.2. The speech signal source is placed in front of the array at a distance of 0.5 m. Two types of noise were used for experiments: Gaussian white noise and engine recorded noise. The white noise was uniformly added at different SNR over each microphones, while engine noise source was placed at a distance of 1 m behind the last microphone of the array.

The signals received through the microphones were applied to a fixed DS beamformer designed to enhance the direction of the desired speech source. For multi-band spectral over-subtraction we used nonlinear frequency spacing with a number of 4 bands that gives an optimal speech quality [7].

Objective and subjective quality evaluation methods were applied to establish the performance of the algorithms presented in this study. In Table 1 the simulations show that the Mean Opinion Score (MOS) computed from ITU-T Recommendation P.862 (PESQ) [8] is increasing when using more than two microphones. Increasing the number of microphones more than four does not give an increasing of quality.

**Table 1.** PESQ MOS evaluation for the enhanced speech.

| Input SNR | Output of the DS beamformer | Bark spaced four multi-band spectral over-subtraction | | | | |
|---|---|---|---|---|---|---|
| Number of microphones | | 2 | 3 | 4 | 5 | 6 |
| 0 dB | 1.75 | 1.79 | 1.82 | 1.85 | 1.84 | 1.84 |
| 5 dB | 1.85 | 1.90 | 1.99 | 1.97 | 1.98 | 1.97 |
| 10 dB | 2.26 | 2.41 | 2.44 | 2.46 | 2.45 | 2.40 |
| 15 dB | 2.82 | 2.86 | 2.88 | 2.90 | 2.89 | 2.84 |

Subjective listening tests indicate that, using the fixed DS beamforming followed by non-linear Bark spaced multi-band over-subtraction, a very good speech quality with less musical noise and with minimal speech distortion is obtained.

Figure 2 shows the spectrogram for speech signal "The sky this morning was clear and light blue" affected by car engine noise, at a SNR of 10 dB at the output of the DS beamformer and the spectrogram of the enhanced speech obtained using over-subtraction with four non-linear Bark spaced bands.

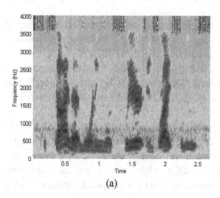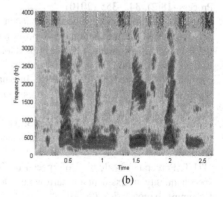

(a)                                                  (b)

**Fig. 2.** Spectrogram of speech signal "The sky this morning was clear and light blue" affected by car noise (a) at the output of the DS beamformer (b) after the multi-band spectral over-subtraction was applied (Color figure online)

## 5  Conclusions

This paper presents an improved noise reduction system using multi-microphone signal processing and a spectral subtraction method that takes into account the non-uniform effect of colored noise on the speech spectrum. The proposed method uses a nonlinear frequency spacing approach for multi-band over-subtraction factor estimation. This compensates the fact that the beamformers will not filter the noise for different frequencies since the beamwidth decreases as frequency increases.

The proposed method also reduces the residual musical tones that appear in the case of conventional power spectral subtraction. Simulations with different types of noise and different configurations for microphone arrays show a better quality for the enhanced speech when using the multi-band spectral subtraction method after the multi-microphone signal processing.

**Acknowledgment.** This work was supported by a grant of the Romanian National Authority for Scientific Research and Innovation, CNCS – UEFISCDI, project number PN-II-RU-TE-2014-4-1880.

## References

1. Berouti, M., Schwartz, R., Makhoul, J.: Enhancement of speech corrupted by acoustic noise. In: Proceedings of the IEEE International Conference on Acoustics, Speech and Signal Processing, pp. 208–211, April 1979
2. Benesty, J., Chen, J., Huang, Y.: Microphone Array Signal Processing. Springer, Heidelberg (2007). https://doi.org/10.1007/978-3-540-78612-2
3. Souden, M., Chen, J., Benesty, J., Affes, S.: An integrated solution for online multichannel noise tracking and reduction. IEEE Trans. Audio Speech Lang. Process. 19(7), 2159–2169 (2011)
4. Cornelis, B., Doclo, S., van dan Bogaert, T., Moonen, M., Wouters, J.: Theoretical analysis of binaural multimicrophone noise reduction techniques. IEEE Trans. Audio Speech Lang. Process. 18(2), 342–355 (2010)
5. Udrea, R.M., Ciochina, S.: Speech enhancement using spectral over-subtraction and residual noise reduction. In: International Symposium on Signals, Circuits and Systems, pp. 165–169. IEEE Press, Iasi, Romania (2003). https://doi.org/10.1109/SCS.2003.1226974
6. Kamath, S., Loizou, P.: A multi-band spectral subtraction method for enhancing speech corrupted by colored noise. In: IEEE International Conference on Acoustics, Speech, and Signal Processing (ICASSP). IEEE Press, Orlando (2002). https://doi.org/10.1109/ICASSP.2002.5745591
7. Udrea, R.M., Vizireanu, N., Ciochina, S., Halunga, S.: Nonlinear spectral subtraction method for colored noise reduction using multi-band Bark scale. Sig. Process. 88(5), 1299–1303 (2008)
8. ITU-T, Perceptual evaluation of speech quality PESQ, an objective method for end-to-end speech quality assessment of narrowband telephone networks and speech codecs, ITU-T Recommendation P.862 (2000)

# Practical Implementation Aspects of the Data Timed Sending (DTS) Protocol Using Wake-up Radio (WuR)

Konstantin Chomu[1]($\boxtimes$), Vladimir Atanasovski[1], Liljana Gavrilovska[1],
and Michele Magno[2,3]

[1] Faculty of Electrical Engineering and Information Technologies,
Ss. Cyril and Methodius University in Skopje,
RugjerBoshkovik 18, 1000 Skopje, Macedonia
{konstantin.chomu,vladimir,liljana}@feit.ukim.edu.mk
[2] D-ITET, ETH Zurich, Gloriastrasse 35, 8092 Zurich, Switzerland
michele.magno@iis.ee.ethz.ch
[3] DEI, University of Bologna, Viale del Resorgimento 2, 40132 Bologna, Italy
michele.magno@unibo.it

**Abstract.** The energy efficient Data Timed Sending (DTS) protocol enables information transfer from sensor nodes to sink host by choosing the appropriate transmission time of a short packet without data payload. Wake-up Radio (WuR) devices allow asynchronous communication of Wireless Sensor Networks (WSNs) putting the sensor nodes' main radio modules in continuous sleep state thus increasing energy efficiency. A common characteristic for the DTS protocol and WuR is that they are designed for applications where sensors take sparse measurements, typically one measurement every few minutes. This paper investigates the combination of the DTS protocol with WuR into a single integrated solution. The analytical analysis shows that the DTS protocol significantly reduces the energy consumption when coupled with WuR making this solution suitable for applications with battery powered WSN (e.g. body area WSN).

**Keywords:** DTS · WuR · WSN · Energy efficiency

## 1 Introduction

Wireless Sensor Networks (WSNs) consist of a number of sensor nodes that wirelessly transfer some measured information to a so-called sink node for further processing. A development bottleneck of WSNs and associated applications is the limited battery power supply of the sensor nodes. The battery lifetime can be prolonged with energy efficient communication protocols and with low-power hardware.

Communication protocols save energy by efficient routing, packet formatting, data processing or other algorithmic solutions. The *Data Timed Sending* (DTS) communication protocol [1–3] achieves energy savings of 25–30% in the sensor nodes, compared with traditional WSN protocols (e.g. ZigBee, LoWPAN etc.), by reducing the packets' size so that the TX radio module spends minimal time in on-state. The very short information to be transferred is coded into the *time* when it is sent rather than in a

© ICST Institute for Computer Sciences, Social Informatics and Telecommunications Engineering 2018
N. Oliver et al. (Eds.): MindCare 2016/Fabulous 2016/IIoT 2015, LNICST 207, pp. 139–144, 2018.
https://doi.org/10.1007/978-3-319-74935-8_20

classical data payload. This allows reduction of the DTS packets to minimal values (no payload needed) at the expense of introducing additional delays in the network.

Traditional WSNs require wake up in regular time intervals (duty-cycling) to listen to the channel. The energy waste caused by continuous channel listening can be significantly lowered using the *Wake-up Radio* (WuR) concept [4–6]. In WuR systems, the sensor node is in continuous sleep-state and an additional always-on ultra low-power receiver, called *Wake-up Radio receiver* (WuRx), is added. The WuRx serves only to detect *Wake-up Call* (WuC), transmitted by the sink node's *Wake-up Transmitter* (WuTx), and to wake up the node after that, whereas the data messages are exchanged through the nodes' main radios in traditional fashion (Bluetooth, ZigBee, etc.). The WuC consists of only a few bytes and contains the destination address that enables selective awakening. WuR system saves energy at sensor nodes.

This paper proposes implementation of the DTS protocol combined with WuR hardware in order to improve the energy efficiency of the WSN communication. Section 2 gives the related work to the DTS operational principle and to WuR. Section 3 presents the integration of the DTS protocol with WuR into a single solution called DTS-WuR that is then compared to the case when no DTS is used. Section 4 gives the results for the energy saving achieved by the DTS-WuR, and, finally, Sect. 5 summarizes the conclusions.

## 2  Related Work on DTS and WuR

The DTS protocol [1–3] formats the time into frames divided into slots and each slot is additionally divided into subslots. Each slot in the frame corresponds to certain sensor node and each subslot corresponds to certain value of the measured phenomenon. The sensor nodes are synchronized with the sink node and the information about the measured value is transferred from the sensor node to the sink node by choosing appropriate time slot and subslot in which the DTS packet will be sent. Due to the communication delay, this protocol is feasible for applications with low measurement rates.

At the hardware level, all components strive to achieve lower energy consumption by ability to work in high and low power modes. The energy saving element in WuR systems is the ultra-low power WuRx that has current consumption in the order of μA or even nA [4]. There are several types of WuR systems [5] such as *in-band* WuRs, *out-of-band* WuRs etc. [7].

Unlike previous works, this paper discusses the implementation aspects of the DTS protocol combined with WuR systems into a single solution. To showcase the benefits of the DTS and WuR combination, the paper additionally performs a comparative energy consumption and energy savings analysis between:

- The combined **DTS-WuR solution**, where the data from the sensor nodes is coded into the exact time when it is sent (inherently introducing additional communication delay in the WSN) and the packets are extremely short with no need for data payload and

- The **no-DTS-WuR solution**, where the data from the sensor nodes is sent imme-
diately upon reception of a WuC with no additional delays, but with a need for
packets with long data payloads.

The rationale behind is that the WuR systems introduce asynchronous WSN
operation, thus comparisons are sound only for cases with and without DTS.

## 3 Practical Implementation of DTS Using WuR

DTS protocol and WuR systems are both suitable for applications with low measurement rates. Their main difference is that the DTS protocol needs synchronization,
whereas the WuR is designed to enable an asynchronous communication. To allow the
integration of the DTS protocol with WuR, the classical DTS protocol [1] undergoes
two modifications:

- Substitution of the continuous nodes' synchronization with temporary synchronization that lasts only during the measurement process and
- Transmission of the DTS packet by the sensor node's WuTx instead of the main
radio transceiver. Since the DTS packet does not contain any data payload, its
length and format are the same as those of WuC and this packet is called Wake-up
Information Message (WuIM). The only difference between the WuIM and WuC is
the content of their destination field.

Figure 1 shows the Message Sequence Chart (MSC) for comparison of the
DTS-WuR system with the no-DTS-WuR system. In the DTS-WuR system, when the
sink node decides to retrieve measurement from a certain sensor node, it wakes up both
its main Micro-Controller Unit (MCU) and WuTx and sends WuC with address code
corresponding to that sensor node. Then, its WuTx goes back into sleep-state.
Simultaneously with the WuC transmission, sink's WuRx starts its stopwatch and the
main MCU goes back into sleep-state. When the response (WuIM) from the sensor
node arrives, sink's WuRx stops the stopwatch, wakes up the main MCU and forwards
the value of time elapsed. Finally, according to the value of time elapsed, the main
MCU calculates the value of the measured phenomenon, stores that value in memory
and goes into sleep-state again.

At DTS-WuR system, before the measurement startup, the sensor node's main
MCU is in sleep-state. When the sensor node's WuRx (which is in on-state all the time)
receives a WuC, it makes address check up and, if the address matches, it wakes up the
main MCU. The main MCU captures the sensor's reading, calculates the waiting time
(delay) and goes back into sleep-state. After the expiration of the waiting time, the main
MCU and WuTx wake up, WuTx sends WuIM with address code corresponding to the
sink node, and then both main MCU and WuTx go back into sleep-state again.

Since the sink's WuRx in the DTS-WuR system spends much less energy than the
sink's RX in the no-DTS-WuR, the DTS-WuR system achieves better energy efficiency
on the sink's side.

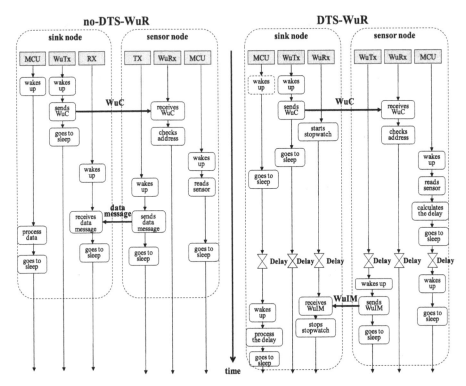

**Fig. 1.** Message Sequence Chart (MSC) for one measurement cycle for the no-DTS-WuR system and for the DTS-WuR system

## 4  Energy Consumption Analysis and Results

The energy consumption comparison between the DTS-WuR and the no-DTS-WuR solution relies on the WuR board presented in [5]. The main energy consumption entities of this 3 V battery powered board are the CC1101 868 MHz transceiver (RX, TX, WuTx) and the MSP430F2350 chip (node's main MCU).

The energy consumption analysis is conducted by calculating the amount of energy the RX, TX, WuRx, WuTx and main MCU (the elements in Fig. 1 plus the sensor) cumulatively spend during one measurement cycle. The power consumption of hardware components, durations of messages, durations of power-mode states, and application parameters are given in Tables 1, 2 and 3.

**Table 1.** Energy consumption parameters for the no-DTS-WuR solution only

| Parameter | Value |
|---|---|
| Main radio power consumption in RX/TX/sleep states | 56.4 mW/52.2 mW/0.6 µW |
| Data message duration | 3.2 ms |

**Table 2.** Energy consumption parameters for the DTS-WuR only

| Parameter | Value |
|---|---|
| WuIM duration | 12.2 ms |

**Table 3.** Energy consumption parameters for both no-DTS-WuR and DTS-WuR solutions

| Parameter | Value |
|---|---|
| Main MCU power consumption in wake-up/sleep states | 900 µW/0.3 µW |
| WuTx power consumption in transmitting/sleep states | 43.2 mW/0.6 µW |
| WuRx power consumption in receiving/idle states | 26.4 µW/7.8 µW |
| WuRx power consumption when transfers data to main MCU | 26.4 µW |
| WuC duration | 12.2 ms |
| WuRx to main MCU data transfer duration | $\approx 0$ s |
| Time needed main MCU to process data | $\approx 31.25$ µs |
| Sensor's power consumption/reading duration | 60 mW/0.5 s |
| Measurement interval | 15 to 120 s |

The sensor power consumption and sensor reading time are set to 60 mW and 0.5 s, respectively, which are common values for WSN sensors. Furthermore, the measurement time interval $T_M$ (time between two successive measurements) is simulated to be in the range of 15 to 120 s. For example, in the body area networks, parameters which can be measured at such rates are body temperature, pulse rate etc.

Figure 2 shows the resulting sink's energy consumption ratio between the no-DTS-WuR ($E_{S-R}$) and the DTS-WuR ($E_{S-D}$). It is evident that the DTS-WuR provides significant energy savings that are higher for smaller measurement intervals.

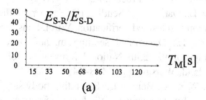

(a)

**Fig. 2.** Sink node energy consumption ratio between no-DTS-WuR and DTS-WuR ($E_{S-R}/E_{S-D}$) for different measurement intervals $T_M$

The comparison of the energy consumption between the traditional TX and the WuTx must take into account both the packet sizes and bit rates. The packet size of the WuIM is considerably lower than the size of the data message, but the WuTx has considerably lower bit rate than the TX as well [5] (due to the lower sensitivity of the WuRx). The power consumptions and durations in the on-state of the TX and the WuTx are such that there is no significant energy saving on the sensor nodes' side. However, there are significant energy savings in the sink.

Typical application scenario where combination of WuR and DTS can show their energy-efficiency would be a body area network where the sink node is battery powered and it retrieves measurements from the remote sensors each 120 s. In this scenario, the WuR hardware alone achieves significant energy savings in the sensor nodes compared to the classical WSNs. But this paper shows that DTS protocol enables the WuR hardware to achieve significant energy savings (20 times) in the sink node too, compared to the classical WSNs.

## 5 Conclusion

This paper combines the DTS protocol with WuR to achieve asynchronous DTS that increases the energy efficiency in WSNs. The DTS protocol codes data into time inherently introducing communication delays. But, the introduction of the DTS protocol allows communication with very short packets significantly increasing the energy efficiency in the WSN. Due to the fact that WuRx consumes much less energy than RX, the energy savings occur at sink nodes making the DTS-WuR suitable for applications with battery powered WSNs.

Future work will comprise experimentation with different parameters and different scenarios (e.g. multiple sensor nodes competing for the medium etc.).

**Acknowledgement.** This work was performed within the SNF project ERT-SEE (IZ74Z0_160481). The authors would like to thank everyone involved.

## References

1. Chomu, K., Gavrilovska, L.: Data Timed Sending (DTS) - energy efficient WSN protocol for smart environmental monitoring. In: Proceedings of ETAI 2013, Ohrid, Macedonia (2013)
2. Chomu, K., Gavrilovska, L.: Data Timed Sending (DTS) energy efficient protocol for wireless sensor networks: simulation and testbed verification. Wirel. Sens. Netw. **5**(8), 158–167 (2013)
3. Chomu, K., Gavrilovska, L.: Data-timed sending method – solution for higher energy efficiency. In: Proceedings of the 25th National Symposium of Telecommunications and Computer Networks, Poland, Warsaw, pp. 1488–1497 (2009)
4. Gomez, A., Magno, M., Wen, X., Benini, L.: Extending body sensor nodes' lifetime using a wearable Wake-up Radio. In: Atanasovski, V., Leon-Garcia, A. (eds.) FABULOUS 2015. LNICST, vol. 159, pp. 108–117. Springer, Cham (2015). https://doi.org/10.1007/978-3-319-27072-2_14
5. Oller, J., Demirkol, I., Casademont, J., Paradells, J., Gamm, G.U., Reindl, L.: Performance evaluation and comparative analysis of SubCarier modulation Wake-up Radio systems for energy-efficient wireless sensor network. Sensors **14**, 22–51 (2014)
6. Magno, M., Benini, L.: An ultra low power high sensitivity Wake-Up Radio receiver with addressing capability. In: 10th IEEE International Conference on Wireless and Mobile Computing, Networking and Communications, Larnaca, Cyprus, pp. 92–99 (2014)
7. Magno, M., Jelicic, V., Srbinovski, B., Bilas, V., Popovici, E., Benini, L.: Design, implementation, and performance evaluation of a flexible low-latency nanowatt Wake-Up Radio receiver. IEEE Trans. Ind. Inform. **12**(2), 633–644 (2016)

# Intrusion Prevention System Evaluation for SDN-Enabled IoT Systems

Alexandru Stancu, Stefan-Ciprian Arseni, Alexandru Vulpe(✉),
Octavian Fratu, and Sinoma Halunga

University Politehnica of Bucharest, 060042 Bucharest, Romania
{alex.stancu,stefan.arseni,alex.vulpe}@radio.pub.ro,
shalunga@elcom.pub.ro

**Abstract.** As the importance of communication networks increases in our lives, the limitations of traditional networks start to emerge. Software Defined Networking (SDN) is the most recent paradigm in the networking industry, its purpose being to mitigate traditional network limitations, such as complexity, the difficulty of introducing new services in the network, the inability of enforcing security policies while having a network-wide view. From a security point of view, the need for middleboxes in the network, such as firewalls or Intrusion Detection/Prevention Systems (IDS/IPS) is eliminated by implementing these functionalities in software applications. As SDN has the potential of becoming a key enabler for the Internet of Things (IoT), there are specific aspects of security for IoT that need to be taken into account, for example the lack of powerful computing resources or limited battery life, making securing IoT devices more challenging. This paper addresses one of these security issues, while evaluating a simple IPS application for an SDN controller. An emulated IoT network is controlled by the SDN controller, which also runs an IPS application. When a node becomes faulty or it is compromised and it sends too much traffic, that could cause a Denial of Service (DoS) in the network, it is blocked by the controller for a configurable amount of time.

**Keywords:** Security · Wireless Sensor Networks
Intrusion detection · Software Defined Networking
Internet of Things

## 1 Introduction

Software Defined Networking (SDN) and Internet of Things (IoT) are two of the most popular recent paradigms in the research community. IoT represents the interconnection of physical items (devices, vehicles, buildings, appliances) that are capable of network connectivity in order to collect and exchange data. SDN is an emerging architecture that decouples the network data plane from the control plane making the network control directly programmable through software

© ICST Institute for Computer Sciences, Social Informatics and Telecommunications Engineering 2018
N. Oliver et al. (Eds.): MindCare 2016/Fabulous 2016/IIoT 2015, LNICST 207, pp. 145–150, 2018.
https://doi.org/10.1007/978-3-319-74935-8_21

applications and abstracting the underlying infrastructure for the network services and applications. It appeared as a solution for mitigating the limitations that traditional networks have proven, such as complexity, vendor dependency, network policies that are not consistent, difficult network management [1].

SDN is beginning to become a key enabler for new concepts, such as IoT, or Cloud Computing, because it satisfies their needs, such as dynamic network reconfiguration, demand of higher bandwidth or simplified network architectures that ease innovation [2].

Functions previously obtained through middle-boxes could be achieved in software applications that run on top of the SDN controller. This has been demonstrated in [3], where an IPS application was implemented for the POX SDN controller.

An example of architecture for security in SDN-enabled IoT networks is defined in [4]. The authors describe how the security of each domain can be enhanced and how to distribute the security rules in order not to compromise the security of one domain in the case of multiple interconnected domains. However they provide no experimental evaluation of their architecture.

Authors in [5] define a SDN architecture for IoT based on Object Management Group's data distribution service (DDS) middleware. They do not, however, study security aspects for this architecture. Finally, the combination of Software Defined Wireless Networking (SDWN) and Wireless Sensor Networks is evaluated against popular networks such as ZigBee and 6LoWPAN in [6]. Authors perform extensive campaign measurements on the EuWin platform, but they evaluate only the protocol stacks of the three solutions, and do not take security into account.

The paper is organized as follows: Sect. 2 presents security aspects that are specific to SDN, IoT and the combination of these two concepts. Section 3 presents the methodology that was used for deploying and evaluating an IPS application for an emulated SDN-enabled IoT system, while Sect. 4 presents and analyses the obtained results. Section 5 highlights the impact of the results and possible future research directions, drawing the conclusions.

## 2    Security Aspects in SDN and IoT

As far as security is concerned, Software Defined Networking has both advantages and disadvantages. A major advantage is that it enables enhanced network security by its ability to redirect or filter traffic flows based on content or network states. The major disadvantage is that SDN is more vulnerable to threats because of the existence of the logically centralized controller.

On the other hand, the rise of the Internet of Things brings about numerous security issues, caused by humans' ever increasing reliance on intelligent devices in most aspects of their lives. These become subject to attacks and intrusions that have the ability to compromise personal privacy or threaten public safety. Such concerns have been addressed in multiple scientific papers that present different views on how IoT security issues have been or are being resolved, but also on key problems that security for IoT needs to address for IoT to become a dependable concept [7–9].

Through the integration of SDN in IoT systems, a part of the security concerns can be addressed, as presented in [10]. By allowing a high level of customization, SDN has become a key concept in the implementation process and also in the evolution of IoT systems [11].

# 3  Methodology

In mininet, a simple tree-like IoT topology was emulated. It contains four Office Gateways, each having five types of sensors. The traffic from every other two Office Gateways is aggregated into a Floor Gateway and then every other two Floor Gateways are aggregated into a Company Gateway. In mininet, the sensors are represented as hosts, and the gateways are considered to be switches (emulated as Open Virtual Switches). ONOS was chosen as the SDN controller for the network, based on several reasons, as described in [12].

Next, an application for ONOS, representing a simple IPS was implemented. Every five seconds, the controller polls through the OpenFlow protocol, the port stats for every device and if traffic passed through a specific port, the IPS application will compute the amount of throughput it received from the host, in kbps. It will then compare that value with a chosen threshold value of 225 kbps, considering a normal traffic pattern of 125 kbps for each host. If the value exceeds that threshold, then a flow rule is installed on the device, dropping all traffic from that port, having a timeout of 60 s, giving the attacked server a good amount of time to process the traffic that was sent until the node was considered malicious. This behavior simulates an IPS.

The third step in the methodology was evaluating the application. Iperf3 was used for generating traffic between the sensors and the server. Three phases of evaluating the application were considered. The first phase consisted in running the mininet topology and connecting it to the ONOS controller, without the IPS application enabled. An iperf3 server was started on the host connected to the Company Gateway, referred to as "Server". After that, an iperf3 client was started on each of the sensors, transmitting UDP traffic to the server, with a throughput of 125 kbps, for a period of 60 s. Also, ping was started from each of the hosts to the Server. Average RTT and jitter were measured by the ping, as well as the jitter and packet loss by the iperf3 server. These values were used to see the normal behavior of the network. The second phase of testing consisted in taking the same measurements, without the IPS application running on the ONOS controller. This time, eight of the sensors were considered to be malicious, and this situation was simulated by sending traffic with a rate of 250 kbps from those hosts. The third phase was identical to the second one, except for the IPS application, that was enabled in the SDN controller.

## 4    Experimental Results

Several network parameters were considered for evaluating the application: the average RTT of the ICMP packets from the sensors to the Server and the standard deviation of the latency for that type of traffic, as measured by the ping tool. Also, the jitter, as measured by the iperf3 client was taken into account.

The ping results from the compromised nodes reveal the amount of time needed by the IPS application to detect the malicious traffic and block it. In ten of the twelve cases, the ping stops after 10 s, and in the other two cases it stops after 15 s. This means an average value of 11.25 s until the faulty node is blocked from the network. The parameters measured with the iperf3 tool highlight other aspects of the traffic in the network. The jitter of the UDP traffic between the clients and the Server increases in 58% of the cases. Such increases of the jitter can drastically affect the performance of the network. After the IPS application is enabled in the ONOS controller and the same tests are conducted, an improvement is observed. In the case of the jitter, the affected nodes percentage decreases to 33%.

The RTT and jitter variations in time are presented in Figs. 1 and 2. For each graphic, three situations were presented: (a) normal traffic conditions, malicious traffic present in the network while the IPS application is disabled and malicious traffic while the IPS application is enabled.

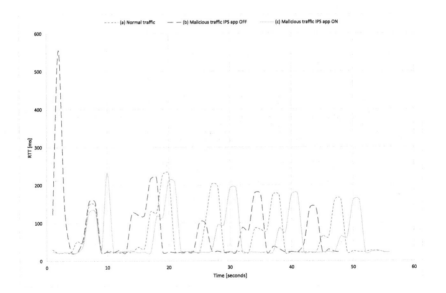

**Fig. 1.** RTT variation

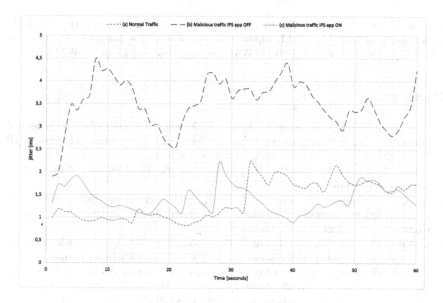

**Fig. 2.** Jitter variation

## 5    Conclusion

Software defined networking is proving to become an important enabler for a rapid and safe implementation of the Internet of Things paradigm. Although the flexibility that SDN brings improves the easiness of integrating dynamically configurable security solutions, there are still issues that need to be addressed.

Through this paper we made an assessment on the performance variation of an SDN-enabled IoT topology, when integrating an IPS application. The simple yet relevant implementation lead to some results that can be applied even for a more comprehensive simulation of a larger IoT system topology. We can state that the basic discovery and control information transmitted throughout the network was not affected by the occurence of some faulty nodes, but there was a drop in performance for the overall network, when faulty nodes were activated. After enabling the IPS application, the drop in performance lasted for a short period of time that would not create an accentuated ripple effect throughout the network.

In conclusion, even simple SDN security applications with a customizable implementation can ensure a minimum level of protection for a network. By integrating the SDN security principle, the internal network is assured with a sufficient level of confidentiality and integrity of data.

**Acknowledgments.** This work has been funded by University Politehnica of Bucharest, through the "Excellence Research Grants" Program, UPB – GEX. Identifier: UPB–EXCELENTA–2016 project "Platform for Studying Security in IoT", contract number 96/2016 (PaSS-IoT), by UEFISCDI Romania under grants no. 20/2012

"Scalable Radio Transceiver for Instrumental Wireless Sensor Networks - SaRaT-IWSN" and 262EU/2014 eWALL support project and by the European Commission by FP7 IP project no. 610658/2013 "eWALL for Active Long Living - eWALL".

# References

1. Stancu, A., Halunga, S., Suciu, G., Vulpe, A.: An overview study of software defined networking. In: 2015 14th International Conference on Informatics in Economy (IE 2015), Bucharest, pp. 50–55, 30 April–3 May 2015
2. Vilata, R., Munoz, R., Casellas, R., Martinez, R.: Enabling internet of things with software defined networking. CTTC (2015)
3. Akin, G., Karaarslan, E., Bük, O., Uçar, E.: SDN architecture fundamentals and DOS prevention basics: a case study with openflow. In: International Scientific Conference, UNITECH 2015, Gabrovo (2015)
4. Flauzac, O., González, C., Hachani, A., Nolot, F.: SDN based architecture for IoT and improvement of the security. In: 2015 IEEE 29th International Conference on Advanced Information Networking and Applications Workshops (WAINA), Gwangiu, pp. 688–693 (2015). https://doi.org/10.1109/WAINA.2015.110
5. Hakiri, A., Berthou, P., Gokhale, A., Abdellatif, S.: Publish/subscribe-enabled software defined networking for efficient and scalable IoT communications. IEEE Commun. Mag. **53**(9), 48–54 (2015). https://doi.org/10.1109/MCOM.2015.7263372
6. Buratti, C., et al.: Testing protocols for the internet of things on the EuWIn platform. IEEE Internet Things J. **3**(1), 124–133 (2016). https://doi.org/10.1109/JIOT.2015.2462030
7. Jing, Q., Vasilakos, A.V., Wen, J., Jingwei, L., Qiu, D.: Security of the Internet of Things: perspectives and challenges. Wirel. Netw. **20**(8), 2481–2501 (2014)
8. Sicaria, S., Rizzardia, A., Griecob, L.A., Coen-Porisinia, A.: Security, privacy and trust in Internet of Things: the road ahead. Comput. Netw. **76**, 146–164 (2015)
9. Nguyen, K.T., Laurent, M., Oualha, N.: Survey on secure communication protocols for the Internet of Things. Ad Hoc Netw. **32**, 17–31 (2015)
10. Olivier, F., Carlos, G., Florent, N.: New security architecture for IoT network. Procedia Comput. Sci. **52**, 1028–1033 (2015)
11. Martinez-Julia, P., Skarmeta, A.F.: Empowering the Internet of Things with software defined networking. In: White Paper, IoT6 - FP7 European research project (2014)
12. Stancu, A., Halunga, S., Vulpe, A., Suciu, G., Fratu, O., Popovici, E.C.: A comparison between several software defined networking controllers. In: 12th International Conference on Advanced Technologies, Systems and Services in Telecommunications (TELSIKS 2015), Niš, Serbia, pp. 223–226, 14–17 October 2015

IIoT 2015

# A Privacy Scheme for Monitoring Devices in the Internet of Things

Zygmunt J. Haas[1(✉)] and Ashkan Yousefpour[2]

[1] Wireless Networks Laboratory, Cornell University, Ithaca, NY 14853, USA
zhaas@cornell.edu
[2] Department of Computer Science, University of Texas at Dallas,
Richardson, TX 75080, USA
ashkan@utdallas.edu

**Abstract.** Sufficiently strong security and privacy mechanisms are prerequisite to amass the promising benefits of the IoT technology and to incorporate this technology into our daily lives. This paper introduces a novel approach to privacy in networks, an approach which is especially well matched with the IoT characteristics. Our general approach is based on continually changing the identifying attributes of IoT nodes. In particular, the scheme proposed in this work is based on changing the IoT nodes' IP addresses, and because the changing patterns of the IP addresses appear random to a non-intended observer, an adversary is unable to identify the source or destination of a particular transmission. Thus, packets that carry information generated by a particular node cannot be linked together. The scheme offers additional security benefits, including DoS mitigation, is relatively easy to implement, and requires no changes to the existing networking infrastructure. We discuss the details of the implementation of the scheme and evaluate its performance.

**Keywords:** Privacy · Anonymity · IoT · Security · IP address hopping

## 1 Introduction and Motivation

To amass the promising benefits of the Internet of Things (IoT) technology, a number of technical challenges have to be overcome, with security being a major such a challenge. Without sufficient degree of security and privacy of information, users will not adopt this new trend that promises to intimately integrate into their lives. It is generally believed that security of Internet of Things is a significantly more challenging problem than the security of today's Internet. First, the number of devices in the IoT increases exponentially and many of these devices will operate unattended, thus more time might pass without a successful attack being detected. Moreover, all the malware that already exists today in the Internet, become viable threats to the small-print IoT devices, incapable of running complex security protection software. Furthermore, a successful attack on IoT devices, such as medical devices, baby-monitoring equipment, smart stove, and house alarm systems, creates potential for severe and immediate danger to their users (e.g., resulting in injury or death), a different type of danger than we are used to with typical Internet malware, such as theft of information.

© ICST Institute for Computer Sciences, Social Informatics and Telecommunications Engineering 2018
N. Oliver et al. (Eds.): MindCare 2016/Fabulous 2016/IIoT 2015, LNICST 207, pp. 153–165, 2018.
https://doi.org/10.1007/978-3-319-74935-8_22

There have been a number of solutions proposed in the literature that preserve privacy for IoT networks (e.g., [1–3]). However, as Internet transmissions require explicit disclosure of source/destination IP addresses, these schemes cannot hide the identity of the IoT nodes, thus allowing the adversaries to learn about the IoT nodes simply by observing the IP addresses in the packets' headers. In contrast, our proposed scheme, aims to actively obfuscate the IP address of a node by allowing the IP address of the node to change frequently (i.e., "IP address hopping"), thus creating uncertainty for adversaries of who is the source/destination of a transmission, while still allowing the packets to be correctly routed to the destination within the Internet.

As an example, consider a hospital facility in which numerous patients are hooked up to medical sensing IoT devices (e.g., EKG, SPO2, GSR, BP, temperature, etc.), together creating an IoT network. The sensors' readings are continuously acquired, packetized, and transmitted to the medical information collection station for processing, archival, and possibly alerting medical personnel of emergency care needed. Such transmissions, being IP-routed, contain the IP addresses of the source device − the IoT sensor of the patient. Typically, such information would also include the identity of the patient. As all the packets originating from the same IoT device would carry the same IP address, an adversary can assemble the medical record of a patient by collecting subsequent packets. In other words, the IP addresses create an index that links all the transmissions together.

Another example could be collection of electricity reading from electric meters. The importance of privacy of such information is well acknowledged, as it could be used by thieves to determine that the house occupants are away and, thus, the house may be subject to a burglary. Of course, a series of readings put together would tell whether the electricity reading decreased in a particular time period, indicative of the occupants being away. Our scheme can preserve the privacy of such information by severing the link between the electricity readings, as well as the readings' link to any ID of a residence.

Using the proposed-here scheme, the IP addresses of subsequent transmissions of each IoT device would be changed in some unpredictable (yet deterministic) pattern, so that the adversary would not be able to use the IP addresses as a linking index of the transmissions. In other words, the adversary will see a massive collection of readings, but will not be able to attribute any reading to a single source (e.g., patient or house, in the previous examples). Of course, the receiver would need to generate a corresponding sequence of the IP addresses, so that the receiver can properly collect together the received information. We further note that, as the pattern of IP addresses is unique to a particular device, there is no need to include the encrypted patient's ID in the packets, as the IP address pattern already identifies a particular IoT device to the receiver (but not to the adversary). In other words, the IP address pattern serves as an ID of the IoT device. Furthermore, an attempt to associate a patient with an IP address of his IoT devices would also be fruitless.

## 2  The Basics of the Scheme

The proposed scheme is useful for information privacy protection in a scenario where a large number of IoT devices transmit similar monitoring (e.g., telemetry) data. More particularly, each transmitted data packet, standing by itself and without association with a particular user, would be useless to an attacker, while either (1) collection of large amount of data coming from a particular user, or (2) association of the data with a particular user, would constitute breach of information privacy. The example of a hospital with large number of the same type of medical sensors would correspond to such a scenario. Similarly, the example of electric meter information from numerous houses in a neighborhood would also present such a scenario.

The basic setup of our scheme includes three nodes, the *IoT node* whose information privacy we intent to protect, the device that communicates with the IoT node, which we refer to as the *corresponding node (CN)*, and a trusted node that controls the operation of the scheme, which we refer to as the *central node*. In a general scenario multiple IoT nodes communicate with multiple corresponding nodes.

The IP address hopping is achieved by a *pseudorandom number generator* that is embedded in a function referred to here as the *Tracking Function (TF)*. The parameters of the *TF* are shared by the IoT node and the authorized CNs. (Note that the *TF* itself does not need to be secret) The *TF* continually generates, what appear to an arbitrary observer, random addresses. We emphasize that although the output of the *TF* seems random, the operation of the function is deterministic; i.e., anyone who observes the output of the *TF*, even for a long time, cannot predict its future values; but whoever holds the *parameters* (including the input) of the *TF* can replicate the output deterministically.

An IoT node uses the random addresses as its actual addresses as they are generated by the *TF*. When an authorized CN desires to communicate with the IoT node, (authorized CN is in possession of the *TF* parameters), it uses the valid (i.e., the current) address generated by the *TF* as the destination address of its transmission. Similarly, transmission from the IoT node uses as the source address the currently generated output based on the *TF*. The IoT node and the CNs generate the IoT node's current IP address every $\zeta$ seconds. Of course, for the scheme to operate properly, some degree of synchronization of the *TF* at the IoT node and the CNs is required – we discuss this in more details later.

The role of the central node is mainly to perform the coordination functions: authenticate the CNs, distribute the TF parameters, and aid in clock synchronization. The central node, the IoT nodes, and the CNs do not have to reside on the same network or even be close to each other. We assume here that the IoT node is static and does not migrate to a new subnet while the scheme is operating, although the scheme could be easily extended to support mobile operation as well.

Our scheme does not introduce additional header information for its operation and it can be incrementally deployed in networks; furthermore, the scheme is compatible with IPv6 addressing. There is no change required for the operation of routing and switching. The required changes to the IP protocol are mostly in the end nodes (the IoT and the CN nodes). If the changes in IP address are sufficiently fast, the scheme could also be used for DoS mitigation at the IoT node.

An alternative scheme would be to implement end-to-end encryption on each of the IoT devices' information flows. Although this would protect the information privacy, we suggest here that the IP address hopping provides significant advantages over encryption. In what follows, we explain why.

If end-to-end encryption were to be implemented, it is clear that multiple keys (probably one key per an IoT device) would need to be maintained. Therefore, some node ID would have to be transmitted in the clear to allow the receiver to choose the proper decryption key. (In fact, the IP address could be such a node ID used to choose the proper key.) As such, the attacker would be able to associate packets with a particular ID, risking loss of privacy. On the other hand, in the proposed scheme, no node ID needs to be transmitted; indeed, even the IP address of the node cannot be interpreted as a node ID, as it is continually changes (even if an attacker is able to associate an IP address with a particular device, such an association would be very short-time living with very limiting privacy consequences). Thus, we maintain that, for the assumed communication scenario, our scheme provides advantageous information privacy scheme, compared with plain encryption.

Furthermore, the proposed scheme avoids the need to maintain the encryption keys and the necessity to periodically rekey the nodes. Finally, the overhead associated with encryption/decryption is eliminated too, which is of particular benefit for resource-constrained devices.

## 2.1   Threat Model

We assume that an adversary can mount passive attacks, such as network scanning and eavesdropping to collect information carried by the packets (including the header information), to assemble information from packets, so as to obtain protected information sent by the IoT nodes (i.e., violating privacy). An attacker can eavesdrop on all connections. In particular, a passive attacker can obtain the current IP address of the IoT node and launch attacks on the IoT node (i.e., becoming an active attacker). We assume that network infrastructure is reliable and not malicious; but may impose delay and packet loss. We further assume that CNs are not malicious and that the central node is a trusted node.

## 2.2   The Tracking Function

In order to generate the IP addresses at the IoT node, we use the timestamp (a sequence that is linearly increasing) as the input to a pseudo-random number generator (PRNG). The timestamp of the IoT node is one of the parameters that is kept secret in our scheme and is in the possession of the secret-sharing nodes. The PRNG, on the other hand, is publicly known; however, without knowing the timestamp and the other parameters the output is unpredictable. In general, any hash function that satisfies the following characteristics, can be used as the scheme's PRNG:

- The function must be one-way secure, meaning that by watching the past values, one cannot guess the parameters of the function.
- The function must be unpredictable; meaning that by watching past values, one cannot predict any future values of the function.
- The function outputs should be randomly distributed on any time scale (at least on a sufficiently long time scale).

The IP address of IoT node is generated by feeding the timestamp to the *Tracking Function*, which is based on PRNG as follows:

$$IP = TF(timestamp) = BA + H_x(timestamp), \qquad (1)$$

where *TF* denotes the *Tracking Function*, *BA* represents the base address of the IoT node's subnet (e.g. '129.110.242.0' without '/24'), and $H_x$ denotes using $x$ least significant bit of the output of the PRNG. $x$ is the minimum number of bits that is required for representing all the available addresses in the IoT node's subnet (*BA* and $x$ can be calculated from the IoT node's subnet address).

We propose to use a chaotic function as the PRNG. In general, chaotic functions are highly sensitive to initial conditions and control parameters, and they appear to behave randomly, alas they are completely deterministic once the set of control parameters is known. A slight change in the input will result in a big change in the output. This property fits well with the goals of the PRNG. More specifically, we use the Hash Function Based on Chaotic Tent Maps as the PRNG of the scheme [4], since it has the aforementioned characteristic. By using the hash function based on a chaotic function, a third-party can neither predict the future values by watching the function, nor generate the function without having the control parameters.

The following is a simple example that demonstrates the operation of the *Tracking Function*. We further assume that we are using IPv4 addressing scheme and that the network address of IoT is 129.110.242.0/24. We need at least 8 bits to represent the

**Table 1.** Output of the *Tracking Function* for 6 samples of timestamp

| Time-stamp | 8 least significant bits of PRNG output | | *Tracking Function* output |
|---|---|---|---|
| | Binary | Decimal | |
| 3000000 | 10000111 | 135 | 129.110.242.135 |
| 3000001 | 00010100 | 20 | 129.110.242.20 |
| 3000002 | 11101100 | 236 | 129.110.242.236 |
| 3000003 | 11111100 | 252 | 129.110.242.252 |
| 3000004 | 00101010 | 42 | 129.110.242.42 |
| 3000005 | 00010010 | 18 | 129.110.242.18 |

host ID portion of the IP address ($x = 8$). Table 1 shows the corresponding generated IP addresses.

Basically, the hash function based on the chaotic tent maps takes in an arbitrary length input $M$ and produces a $2l$-bit hash output, where $l$ is the blocks' size into which the message $M$ is broken. $n$ is the number of rounds in the function. If $M < l$, the block is padded so that the size of the message is a multiple of $l$. In our scheme, the hash function takes in the timestamp as the input M and a pair of initial binary fractions $(s_0, t_0)$, producing a hash output that is a $2l$-bit binary number. Yet we only use the required number of bits ($x$) that is needed to represent all the available IP addresses in a subnet. The initial parameters $(s_0, t_0)$ could be chosen in different ways, but for a good perturbation we use here $(s_0, t_0) = (0.1010...10, 0.0101...01)$. In [4], the author showed that the hash function is resistant to target attack, free-start target attack, collision attack, semi-free-start collision attack, and free-start collision attack, as the computational complexity of these attacks are $2^l$, $2^l$, $2^{l/2}$, $2^{l/2}$, $2^{l/2}$ respectively.

After successful authentication with the central node, authorized CNs get the parameters of the *Tracking Function* from the central node. The parameters are: timestamp, $\zeta$, $l$, and subnet address of the IoT node.

### 2.3   Clock Synchronization

As discussed below, some degree of clock synchronization is required in the scheme to guarantee that timestamps of the central node, the CNs, and the IoT nodes are synchronized. Clock synchronization algorithms sync two or more clocks that have a non-zero drift rate. Typically, drift rate is a very small number; but due to the high frequency of clocks, this can lead to a large difference in clocks even after a short while. The timestamp that we use in our solution, however, is different from the local clock of the operating system. The timestamp that we use is a number that increases by one every $\zeta$ seconds. The central node, after authenticating the CN, performs coarse clock synchronization with the CN, before sending the *Tracking Function* control parameters to the CN. Note that all the nodes (central node, IoT node, and CN), perform clock synchronization periodically.

Let us assume that $\eta$ is the number of times that an IP address changes in each clock synchronization period $\tau$; i.e., $\tau = \zeta \times \eta$, where $\eta$ is a parameter that reflects the accuracy of the clocks in use and is calculated based on the maximum drift rate as follows. Assume that the maximum drift rate in the system is defined by $\delta$ [sec/sec]. Usually $\delta$ is a small number (e.g., $10^{-6}$). The maximum skew between the clocks in the system after 1 s would be $2 \times \delta$ [sec]. We know that timestamp increases by one every $\zeta$ seconds. The maximum skew between two timestamps should be always kept less than one within the interval of clock synchronization (every $\tau$ seconds). This way the timestamps will always be equal, since they are integer numbers. Let $S$ denote the skew between the timestamps within $\tau$ seconds; thus we require that $S < 1$:

$$S = 2 \times \delta \times 1/\zeta \times \tau = 2 \times \delta \times \eta \longrightarrow \eta < \frac{1}{(2 \times \delta)} \tag{2}$$

There are many clock synchronization solutions in the literature that can be used for our scheme (e.g., [5, 6]). For instance, Network Time Protocol (NTP) is a low-cost solution whose accuracy ranges from hundreds of microseconds to several milliseconds [7]. The reference [8] presents a precise relative clock synchronization protocol for distributed applications. It achieves clock precision on the order of 10 μs in small-scale LANs and sub-millisecond over LANs. For our experiment (Sect. 4), we implemented an NTP-like clock synchronization program, where the central node is an NTP server and the other nodes in the system synchronize their clock with it.

## 3  Performance Issues

### 3.1  Address Collision

If many IoT nodes in a subnet use the IP hopping scheme, there is a probability that, at some point in time, two (or more) nodes will be assigned the same IP address. This, of course, is an undesirable situation that should be avoided. In this section, we estimate the probability of such an *address collision*.

Suppose that, in a particular subnet, there are $k + h$ nodes, $k$ of which are IoT nodes and $h$ are other non-IoT nodes (e.g., assigned permanent IP addresses). Further, assume that $m$ is the total number of available IP addresses in the subnet. Then, the probability that two or more IoT nodes will be randomly assigned the same IP address (i.e., the probability of address collision) is:

$$p = 1 - \frac{(m - h) \times (m - h - 1) \times \ldots \times (m - h - k + 1)}{m^k} \tag{3}$$

We assumed that each IP address can be assigned by the *Tracking Function* with equal probability of $1/m$, because the *Tracking Function* is technically based on a pseudo-random number generator, thus the probability of all possible outputs is equal [4]. The author in [4] maintains that for any $0 \leq \alpha < 1$, the distribution of $x_1 = G_\alpha(x_0)$, which is the core of the Hash Function based on Chaotic Tent Maps, for randomly chosen $0 < x_0 < 1$ is the standard uniform distribution, $\mathcal{U}(0, 1)$.

Figure 1 shows the address collision probability as a function of the address space size, $m$, for different values of $k$ and $h$ ($h + k < m < 256$). As shown in the figure, when there are only IoT nodes in the subnet (i.e., $h = 0$), the address collision probability for network sizes of $m > 40$ is negligibly small. When there are 5 normal nodes ($h = 5$) in addition to the active IoT nodes, the address collision probability is not negligible anymore. This provides guidance to the design process of such IoT subnets.

### 3.2  Packets in Transit

As discussed before, due to clock mis-synchronization and intrinsic network delays, packets arriving after a change in IP address has occurred at the IoT node, may still carry the old IP address of the IoT node and, thus, may be discarded at the destination. A mechanism is needed that will prevent or at least minimize the loss of packets in

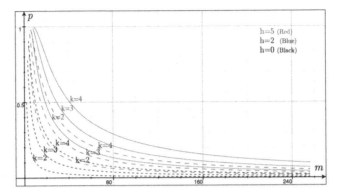

**Fig. 1.** Address collision probability as a function of address range, $m$, with $k$ IoT nodes.

transit during the changes of network addresses. In the approach that we propose here, the IoT node continues to maintain the old IP address (together with the new one) for a short while, so that packets arriving with the old IP address after the IP address has already changed will still be accepted. Of course, the duration of time when both IP addresses are in use should be short to achieve higher privacy in IoT node, as well as to reduce the probability of address collision.

The timing diagram explaining the scheme's operation is presented in Fig. 2. In the upper portion of the diagram presented are the assignments of the IP addresses to the IoT node as a function of time. As we can observe, initially, the IP address of $IP_1$ is

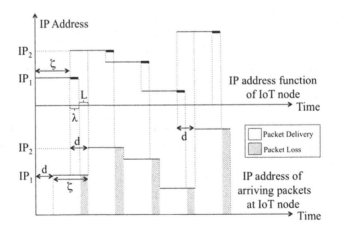

**Fig. 2.** Address possible packet loss due to mismatch of IP addresses. Upper graph: IP address at the IoT node; lower graph: IP address of packets arriving at the IoT node.

assigned to the IoT node and is maintained for the period of $\zeta$, after which time the new $IP_2$ is assigned. However, $IP_1$ is kept active for an additional time $\lambda$ (the thicker line), during which time the IoT node is assigned both $IP_1$ and $IP_2$ addresses.

We now assume that the network introduces delay of $d$ to the packet sent from the CN. The lower portion of Fig. 2 displays the IP addresses of packets arriving at the IoT node. In this example, we assume that the only cause of mis-synchronization of the IP addresses is the network delay (i.e., that the clocks are perfectly synchronized). We see that the IP addresses of packets arriving at the IoT node follow exactly the IP addresses assigned at the IoT node (upper portion of Fig. 2), but they are delayed by $d$. In this example, $\lambda < d$, so some packets arrive at the IoT node after the old IP address, $IP_1$, has already been dropped (after the extra time $\lambda$); such packets are lost (the loss is marked in darker vertical spaces in the lower portion of Fig. 2). It is easy to observe that if $\lambda > d$, then no packet loss would occur. Next, we present a simple analysis of the packet loss.

Let us consider a long time interval $T$ and, for simplicity, assume that $T$ is a multiple of $\zeta$; i.e., $T = c \cdot \zeta$, for some integer $c$. We further assume that the generation rate of packets by the CN is Poisson with rate $\gamma$. Since we assume that the only source of packet loss is the mismatch in IP addresses (i.e., no network losses), the total arrival of packets to the IoT node is also Poisson with rate $\gamma$. Then the average packet loss is:

$$E[Packet\ Loss] = \frac{E[number\ of\ lost\ packets\ in\ the\ interval\ T]}{E[total\ number\ of\ sent\ packets\ in\ the\ interval\ T]} = \frac{E\left[\begin{array}{c} total\ number \\ of\ sent\ packets \\ in\ the\ interval\ T \end{array}\right] - E\left[\begin{array}{c} number\ of \\ received\ packets \\ in\ the\ interval\ T \end{array}\right]}{E[total\ number\ of\ sent\ packets\ in\ the\ interval\ T]}$$

$$= \frac{\gamma \cdot c \cdot \zeta - \gamma \cdot c \cdot (\zeta - \min(0, d - \lambda))}{\gamma \cdot c \cdot \zeta} = \frac{\min(0, d - \lambda)}{\zeta} = \frac{\min(0, L)}{\zeta},$$

$$(4)$$

where we labeled $d - \lambda \equiv L$. Thus, the measure of probability of loss is $L$. To minimize the probability of loss, either $\lambda \cong d$ or $\zeta \gg d - \lambda$. The first case requires the knowledge of the value of $d$, which typically has a non-stationary distribution. Similarly, in the second case, when $d$ is large, it requires either large $\zeta$ or large $\lambda$, leading to limiting degree of achievable privacy. In either case, there is a need for a mechanism to estimate the value of $d$, which can be measured by a one-way delay measurement scheme.

## 3.3 Privacy Protection

The privacy of the scheme primarily relies on the fact that the sequence of the generated IP addresses cannot be predicted neither by anyone who does not possess the parameters of the *Tracking Function*, nor by observing the past sequence of the IP addresses. To test the temporal randomness of a function the standard method is to compute the correlation of the function at various times, i.e., the function's *autocorrelation*. We conducted experimentation with the hash function we used in our scheme, collecting the samples over sufficiently long time to calculate the autocorrelation. The experiment showed white-noise like autocorrelation (an impulse $\delta(x)$ response), demonstrating the lack of correlation in the hash function based on chaotic tent maps.

## 4 Experimentation Results

In this section, we provide some results of the experimental implementation of the scheme. We used three machines as the main components of the scheme. One machine served as the IoT node, one as the central node, and one as the CN that communicated with the IoT node. In order to evaluate the behavior of the basic scheme, we experimented with the scheme over a local-area (UTD, in Richardson, TX) network, as well as over a wide-area network, where the CN resided at Cornell University, in Ithaca, NY. The goal was to understand the performance as a function of different settings of the scheme, with drastically different distributions of the network delays. The results are summarized in Table 2 (local-area network) and Table 3 (wide-area network), for two values of $\lambda = 0.3$ s and $\lambda = 0.8$ s and $\zeta = 1, 2, 3, 4$, and 8 s.

**Table 2.** Packet loss (%) for different values of $\zeta$ and $\lambda$ (Experiment over local-area network)

| (a) $\lambda = 0.3$s | | | | | (b) $\lambda = 0.8$s | | | | |
|---|---|---|---|---|---|---|---|---|---|
| $\zeta$(sec) | 1 | 2 | 3 | 4 | 8 | 1 | 2 | 3 | 4 | 8 |
| Mean | 2.22 | 0.87 | 0.66 | 0.39 | 0.29 | 1.20 | 0.86 | 0.95 | 0.80 | 0.36 |
| 95% CI | [1.93,2.51] | [0.83,0.9] | [0.58,0.73] | [0.35,0.42] | [0.28,0.3] | [1,1.39] | [0.8,0.93] | [0.8,1.07] | [0.66,0.92] | [0.3,0.41] |
| Min | 0.18 | 0.67 | 0.30 | 0.17 | 0.24 | 0.18 | 0.29 | 0.54 | 0.38 | 0.21 |
| Max | 4.09 | 1.16 | 1.31 | 0.58 | 0.37 | 3.08 | 1.92 | 2.11 | 2.07 | 0.87 |

In our implementation, the IoT node resides in a network of size 256. We used the following parameters for the Tracking Function: $l = 16$, $n = 75$, $x = 8$ and $(s_0, t_0) = (0.10101010, 0.01010101)$.

As we can see in Table 2, in local-area networks, for $\zeta > 2$ s, the packet loss is smaller than 1%. To achieve similar packet loss, in the wide-area network, it is required that $\zeta > 4$ s (Table 3). In the experiment in local-area network, most of the losses occur due to delays of running the code, and in particular, due to the delay required for changing the IP addresses in a Linux machine.

**Table 3.** Packet loss (%) for different values of $\zeta$ and $\lambda$ (Experiment over wide-area network)

| (a) $\lambda = 0.3$s | | | | | (b) $\lambda = 0.8$s | | | | |
|---|---|---|---|---|---|---|---|---|---|
| $\zeta$(sec) | 1 | 2 | 3 | 4 | 8 | 1 | 2 | 3 | 4 | 8 |
| Mean | 2.22 | 0.87 | 0.66 | 0.39 | 0.29 | 1.20 | 0.86 | 0.95 | 0.80 | 0.36 |
| 95% CI | [1.93,2.51] | [0.83,0.9] | [0.58,0.73] | [0.35,0.42] | [0.28,0.3] | [1,1.39] | [0.8,0.93] | [0.8,1.07] | [0.66,0.92] | [0.3,0.41] |
| Min | 0.18 | 0.67 | 0.30 | 0.17 | 0.24 | 0.18 | 0.29 | 0.54 | 0.38 | 0.21 |
| Max | 4.09 | 1.16 | 1.31 | 0.58 | 0.37 | 3.08 | 1.92 | 2.11 | 2.07 | 0.87 |

Figure 3 shows the average packet loss for a range of values of the parameter $\zeta$, where $\lambda = 0.2 \cdot \zeta$. This experiment was done both over the LAN at UTD and also over a WAN (where the CN was at Cornell University). The same parameters for the *Tracking Function* were used as before. The figure demonstrates that there is a "threshold" value of $\zeta$, below which the packet loss rapidly increase, while above the threshold the packet loss remains relatively negligible. Thus, as long as $\zeta$ is above the threshold, the packet loss is not much sensitive to the actual value of $\zeta$. In Fig. 3, this threshold is $\zeta = 0.7$ s for the experiment over the local-area network and $\zeta = 1$ s for experiment over the wide-area network.

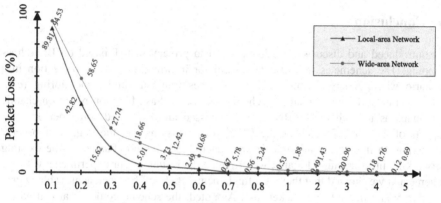

**Fig. 3.** Average packet loss (%) for different $\zeta$ (sec)

## 5  Related Work

There are some related works that use address hopping technique, although either in a different manner or for a different reason. Some of these works are primarily related to the well-known concept of frequency hopping in wireless networks. The works of Shi et al. [9, 10] discusses port and address hopping for active cyber defense (generally DoS). In their work, privacy is not always preserved, as hopping is not done continuously. In their more recent work [11], they presented a scheme that requires Hopping Agent that is responsible for the hopping operation while the security-critical server is hidden behind it. Our approach does not require agent and is more suitable for IoT scenarios where devices are connected in different settings.

Another interesting work based on address hopping is Mirage [12], which is mainly designed for defending against DDoS for web applications. However, the scheme cannot be used for privacy preserving in the IoT, since, the scheme is only activated when under active attack (and only then, it hops every 5 min). Furthermore, it does not match the resource-constrained devices in IoT, as it requires solving puzzles, filtering by routers, and sending large size ACL files (few hundred thousand entries for small attacks) to routers, on each address change.

Similarly, a more recent related work based on address hopping by Krylov et al. [13] addressed DDoS attack mitigation. Their system is not scalable to the IoT networks, since several routers are required (and should support the scheme) to protect a single node. Comparably, the work [14] discusses the general idea of network address hopping, but it is not suited for IoT networks, as much information needs to be sent between two peers each time a communication needs to be established between two nodes. Also their scheme is not scalable to IoT, as the hopping is on per-packet basis (only one-to-one communications is supported). In contrast, in our scheme, only the scheme's parameters (i.e., a few numbers) are transmitted when a new CN joins, and it supports one-to-many communication, namely suitable for IoT.

## 6 Conclusion

We introduced and discussed a scheme for data privacy in IoT based on IP address hopping. The scheme is in particular useful for information privacy protection in a scenario where a large number of IoT devices transmit similar monitoring (e.g., telemetry) data. To implement the scheme, we used a hash function based on chaotic tent maps as the scheme's PRNG. We discussed and evaluated some performance aspects of the scheme, such as the IP address collisions and the degree of privacy protection. In its basic configuration, the scheme requires no changes to the existing networking infrastructure. Finally, we provided the results of our experiments with the scheme and we showed that there is a fundamental trade-off between achievable degree of privacy and the average packet loss. As noted, the scheme could be also used for location-privacy and for protection against DoS attacks. We intend to evaluate these directions in our future work.

**Acknowledgement.** The work of Z. J. Haas has been supported by the NSF grant numbers: CNS-1040689, ECCS-1308208 and CNS-1352880.

## References

1. Beresford, A.R., Stajano, F.: Mix zones: user privacy in location-aware services. In: PERCOMW 2004 Proceedings of the Second IEEE Annual Conference on Pervasive Computing and Communications Workshops, pp. 127–131 (2004)
2. Fan, Y., Lin, B., Jiang, Y., Shen, S.: An efficient privacy-preserving scheme for wireless link layer security. In: IEEE Globecom Wireless Communication Symposium, pp. 4652–4656 (2008)
3. Banerjee, D., Dong, B., Taghizadeh, M., Biswas, S.: Privacy-preserving channel access for Internet of Things. IEEE Internet Things J. **1**, 430–445 (2014)
4. Yi, X.: Hash function based on chaotic tent maps. IEEE Trans. Circuits Syst. II Express Briefs **52**, 354–357 (2005)
5. Mills, D.L.: Internet time synchronization: the network time protocol. IEEE Trans. Commun. **39**, 1482–1493 (1991)
6. Yoon, S., Veerarittiphan, C., Sichitiu, M.L.: Tiny-Sync: tight time synchronization for wireless sensor networks. ACM Trans. Sens. Networks **3**, 1–33 (2007)

7. Mallada, E., Meng, X., Hack, M., Zhang, L., Tang, A.: Skewless network clock synchronization. In: 2013 21st IEEE International Conference on Network Protocols, pp. 1–10 (2013)
8. Tian, G.S., Tian, Y.C., Fidge, C.: Precise relative clock synchronization for distributed control using TSC registers. J. Netw. Comput. Appl. **44**, 63–71 (2014)
9. Shi, L., Jia, C., Lü, S., Liu, Z.: Port and address hopping for active cyber-defense. In: Yang, C.C., et al. (eds.) PAISI 2007. LNCS, vol. 4430, pp. 295–300. Springer, Heidelberg (2007). https://doi.org/10.1007/978-3-540-71549-8_31
10. Shi, L., Jia, C., Lu, S.: DoS evading mechanism upon service hopping. In: 2007 IFIP International Conference on Network and Parallel Computing Workshop, pp. 119–122 (2007)
11. Zhao, C., Jia, C., Lin, K.: Technique and application of End-hopping in network defense. In: 2010 1st ACIS International Symposium on Cryptography, and Network Security, Data Mining and Knowledge Discovery, E-Commerce and Its Applications, and Embedded Systems, pp. 266–270 (2010)
12. Mittal, P., Kim, D., Hu, Y.-C., Caesar, M.: Mirage: towards deployable DDoS defense for web applications. arXiv:1110.1060 (2012)
13. Krylov, V., Kravtson, K.: IP fast hopping protocol design. In: Proceedings of the 10th Central and Eastern European Software Engineering Conference in Russia (2014)
14. Sifalakis, M., Schmid, S., Hutchison, D.: Network address hopping: a mechanism to enhance data protection for packet communications. In: IEEE International Conference on Communications, 2005, ICC 2005, pp. 1518–1523 (2005)

# Short Papers

# How to Deal with Interoperability Testing in the Challenging and Ever-Changing Context of IoT

César Viho[1]([✉]) and Xiaohong Huang[2]

[1] IRISA-University of Rennes 1, Campus de Beaulieu, 35042 Rennes-cedex, France
Cesar.Viho@irisa.fr
[2] BUPT, Beijing 100876, People's Republic of China
huangxh@bupt.edu.cn
http://www.irisa.fr/tipi

**Abstract.** The Internet of Things is a challenging domain for interoperability testing. There are plenty of new standards proposed by the standardization organisations for all levels of the network architecture. Billions of products and applications are developed based on those frequently modified updated standards. This position paper presents means that can help in tackling the problem of interoperability testing of IoT protocols.

**Keywords:** Internet of Things (IoT) · Interoperability testing
Testing initiatives · Tools · Plugtests

## 1 Introduction

Guaranteeing interoperability in the context of Internet of Things (IoT) is tremendously challenging. Here are the main reasons:

- The IoT landscape is large and heterogeneous as it covers several sectors: transportation, healthcare, smart homes/cities, etc. Each of these sectors has their own technologies. This leads to multiple different protocols that will co-exist; increasing by this way the risk of non-interoperability.
- Users are urging companies to provide products and services as soon as the corresponding standards are published. This pressure obliges companies to start developing their products based on the preliminary versions/drafts of those standards.
- Consequently, the testing process is also under pressure. Testing labs can no more wait for the final version of the standard (the RFC in the case of the IETF) to provide associated test suites. It means that test process has to follow the evolution and timeline of the standardization process.

This work has been done in the context of the International Science and Technology Cooperation and Exchange Project of China (2013DFE13130).

© ICST Institute for Computer Sciences, Social Informatics and Telecommunications Engineering 2018
N. Oliver et al. (Eds.): MindCare 2016/Fabulous 2016/IIoT 2015, LNICST 207, pp. 169–170, 2018.
https://doi.org/10.1007/978-3-319-74935-8

- The other issue is the number of components to be tested. It is clearly much more complicated and complex to deal with billions of multi-protocol IoT devices.
- The other big issue is that companies are also trying to reduce time-to-market. They don't want to waist their time in long certification or labelling process.

In this position statement paper, we will give some ingredients that participate in tackling efficiently and successfully these issues. We argue that the three main pilars are:

1. Developing easy-to-use, remotely accessible and easily updatable testing suites and tools
2. Organizing regular interoperability events or Plugtests
3. Providing lightweight certification or labeling processes

To corroborate our statement, we will consider the example of the CoAP (Constrained Application Protocol) developed by the IETF (Internet Engineering Task Force) - CORE (Constrained RESTful Environments) Working Group.

## 2    Content of the Paper

We will first present elements that show the large scope of the Internet of Things. The different types of architecture that can be found in the IoT landscape will be presnted highlighting the increasing risk of non-interoperability. By considering the context of the CoAP protocol, we will describe the evolution of the standardization process from the first drafts to the current drafts or RFCs, including the modifications that have been done till now. We will show how the testing tools have evolved to follow those changes and modifications. The CoAP interoperability events that have been organized and their results will be presented showing their impact on global interoperability achievement. This paper will end by a short discussion on the needs of lightweight certification processes.

# Wi-Suite: Tools and Services for Managing IoT Infrastructures

Alan McGibney[(⊠)] and Susan Rea

Nimbus Centre, Rossa Avenue, Bishopstown, Cork, Ireland
{alan.mcgibney, susan.rea}@cit.ie

**Abstract.** Wi-Suite was developed as a cloud based platform consisting of tools and services to enable users of varying levels of expertise to achieve a reliable wireless sensor network by supporting 3 critical phases of the development lifecycle, design, deploy and management.

**Keywords:** Wireless sensor networks · IoT infrastructure · Smart objects
Support tools and services

## 1 Overview

IoT is billed as a single unifying paradigm to bridge the divide between the digital and physical worlds. While the principle of IoT is simple in terms of understanding the concept the realization of IoT solutions is far more complex. There are a number of challenges faced when designing, deploying and managing IoT solutions that need to be overcome to lower the barrier-to-entry and simplify the exposure of smart objects to IoT services and applications. The appetite for immediate and sustained access to real-time data continues to explode the IoT market size with the expected number of devices to be in the order of billions. While the central focus is on data provisioning the wider implications for managing, monitoring, and maintaining the underlying network infrastructure used to deliver this data, though less obvious, are something that cannot be ignored. Wireless sensors and actuator networks (WSANs) are viewed as a key enabling technology to bridge the gap between the physical and virtual world to realise IoT where IoT offers the ability to interconnect real world objects (RWO) and allow them to interact and cooperate with each other and/or users to form new applications. There are many proprietary and non-proprietary solutions available for WSAN which have led in the development of a static one-to-one relationship between the WSAN devices and the application case. This scenario driven approach has resulted in WSAN becoming information silos with limited connectivity to the external world prohibiting their impact and stifling the large scale deployment of these networks. While these benefits are attractive, to achieve a reliable wireless network is a complex task that requires the installer to consider many influencing factors such as, the dynamic nature of deployment environments, heterogeneity of devices, protocols and middleware, network topology, architectures, lifetime. There remains a significant lack of support for designers, installers and system managers and it is almost a *black art* to create a reliable WSAN. A number of hardware based tools are available that enables an installer to supplement

© ICST Institute for Computer Sciences, Social Informatics and Telecommunications Engineering 2018
N. Oliver et al. (Eds.): MindCare 2016/Fabulous 2016/IIoT 2015, LNICST 207, pp. 171–172, 2018.
https://doi.org/10.1007/978-3-319-74935-8

their experience with a crude indicator of connectivity, while this may be suitable for small scale installations larger deployments in complex RF environments becomes non-trivial. Wi-Suite was developed as a cloud based platform of tools and services to enable users of varying levels of expertise to achieve a reliable wireless sensor network by supporting 3 critical phases of the development lifecycle. The demonstration will showcase the tool suite by providing a walk-through of how the tools and services can be used to support the design, deployment and management of WSAN in the context of a real built environment. Conference delegates will be encouraged to use the tools to design new WSAN deployments and gain insight and understanding of the key considerations for reliable network performance and management.

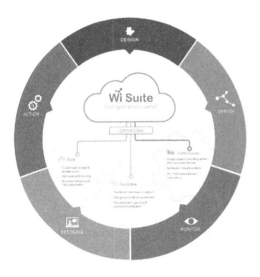

- **Design:** Automatically optimize the number and position of wireless devices, gateways and repeaters to ensure reliable communications and high quality data capture.
- **Deploy:** Tools to make it easy to setup, configure and verify the deployment is operating as it should.
- **Manage:** Services to allow the network to manage itself and pro-actively inform you when action is required.

The authors wish to acknowledge the support of the EU Commission under the FP7 GENiC project (Grant Agreement No 608826) in part funding the work reported in this paper.

# Author Index

Printed in the United States
By Bookmasters